UNSTOPPABLE
HEALTH

7 BREAKTHROUGH HABITS
TO FEEL YOUNGER, GROW STRONGER,
AND ENJOY MORE ENERGY

Dr. Ritamarie Loscalzo
MS, DC, CCN, DACBN

Functional Health Publishing

AUSTIN, TX

Functional Health Publishing
9508 Bell Mountain Drive
Austin, TX 78730
www.drritamarie.com

Book Cover: Jazzy Bulacito
Book Interior: Ambicionz
www.ambicionz.com

Disclaimer

The techniques and advice described in this book represent the opinions of the author based on training and experience. The author expressly disclaims any responsibility for any liability, loss or risk, personal or otherwise, incurred as a result of using any of the techniques, recipes or recommendations suggested herein. If in any doubt, or if requiring medical advice, please contact the appropriate health professional.

Unstoppable Health/ Dr. Ritamarie Loscalzo. — 1st ed.
ISBN 978-1545372890

Praises for Unstoppable Health

"Unstoppable Health is a gift in disguise. You may start reading this book, thinking you will quickly scan through and see what tips you can use in your life that you don't already know about. Prepare for a surprise! This book will take you by the hand from the beginning and ask you to sit down and become involved. You will see so many facets of yourself throughout the book that you will be laughing out loud. The best part of it is that you will realize how easily you can incorporate the ideas into your life. Enjoy the book over and over, especially after you get the recipes!"

Lynn Debuhr Johnson
Health Coach, Homeschooling Mom of 7

"In Unstoppable Health", Dr. Ritamarie Loscalzo goes beyond specious cookie-cutter solutions to provide 7 simple, powerfully effective breakthrough habits that transform your health, happiness, and mindset to transcend ordinary and become lean, sexy, energetic, and authentically tap into your best life. Groundbreaking stuff!"

JJ Virgin

**New York Times Best Selling Author
of The Virgin Diet and The Sugar Impact Diet**

"A realistic and inspirational story about what it really takes to lose weight, get healthy and truly be unstoppable in your life!"

**Michele Pariza Wacek
Best-selling Author of The Love-Based Copywriting
and Marketing Series and The Stolen Twin**

"If you are on a journey seeking more health, energy, and fulfillment, then this book could be your catalyst. I felt like I was the main character in this story. I actually teared up a few times when I was reminded that I am not always living to my full potential. This book will give you hope, clarity and a plan on how to start a new chapter in your own life."

**Keldie Jamieson
Certified Online Business Manager/Owner
Strive Online Solutions**

To my parents, Mary and Rocky, my sister Cathy, my father-in-law Manny, my mother-in-law Naomi, my brother-in-law Michael, my grandparents Rita, Charles, Filomina, and Frank, and all my departed aunts, uncles, cousins, and friends. May you rest in peace, knowing I'm dedicated to sharing life-saving health information with all who are ready to avoid needless pain and suffering, and step into their greatness.

With all my love,

Ritamarie

Acknowledgments

A book like this just wouldn't be possible without the help and inspiration of many people.

Special thanks to my teachers, near and far, living and passed, who inspired, motivated and encouraged me to be my best. The knowledge and experience you've imparted to me has contributed to who I am today.

To my patients and students, whose expressions of delight when they "get it" make all the time and effort worth every minute of my mission. I learn as much from you as you do from me. Thank you from the bottom of my heart.

To Liz Alexander, The Book Doula. She took the ideas that lay deep inside me and helped birth them into the world in written format. The hours we spent thinking, discussing, writing and re-writing resulted in the work you now have in your hands. Without Liz's patience and persistence, expertise and talents, this book would still be but a vision in my head. Liz, I can't thank you enough for your loving support, firm guidance, and amazing ability to transform ideas into a written manuscript.

Special thanks to my dear husband, Scott Claver, who selflessly shares me with the world. Your patience and generosity with my long hours of writing, as well as your diligent care for our children so I can carry out my mission, makes my life so much more fulfilling and purposeful. Thank you from the deepest places in my heart and soul.

And finally, I acknowledge my children, Eric and Kevin, for patiently tolerating a mom who is unlike your friends' Moms.

You've endured my "different" approach to nutrition - and life itself. You've loved and supported me, and above all, adopted most of my ideals and values as your own. You see the world differently from how your friends see it, and you "get" the importance of fresh food, fresh thoughts, and a non-toxic environment. I love you with all my heart.

Table of Contents

Preface

If you're anything like me, you doubtless have tons of self-help and how-to books on your shelves, many of which you've dipped into or skimmed, but rarely read from cover to cover.

New books in the health genre are released every day, so my challenge in writing this was to make sure it stood out - not just in regards to the work I'm known for, but also in comparison to all the other health books out there. Most importantly, I wanted to write a book that would compel readers to devour it completely, to digest it with interest, and eagerly anticipate what comes next.

What better way to do that than by creating fictional characters who would carry my message for me?

It's well-established that people learn best and recall more when taught in story form than through a simple reiteration of facts. People tend to be able to vividly remember the stories later on, whereas facts tend to get "muddied," and are generally more easily forgotten.

I experienced this firsthand when I was homeschooling my kids. We studied a set of books entitled "The Story of the World." It was ancient history retold in story form, with young characters, and I suddenly found myself actually enjoying history, which I'd found boring when I was in school.

The power of story to keep interest and to teach is why I decided to write this first book in story form. There is so much to learn from the experience of others.

The characters in this book are composites of real people. The heroine, Jenny, represents many clients I have counseled over the years. Aunt Sue is a blend of myself and the best mentors I have encountered throughout my almost 30 year career in the health field, counseling people about ways to enhance their health and well-being. The other characters are real people who most of us can recognize from our own lives: the friends who are always there to support us, as well as the ones who feel threatened when we try to change, and want us to stay exactly where we are for their own reasons. Every character in this book represents, in some way, what I learn from my clients as I sit across from them and listen to their stories about their lives, loves, challenges and dreams.

However, my desire was to create more than just a nice story with characters you could relate to and care about. My intent was to incorporate an abundance of useful information to help you actually create positive change in your life, so you can *live better*.

Throughout the book, you'll be exposed to the holistic approach that underpins my entire practice. As you immerse yourself in Jenny's life, my wish is that you take from her transformational journey the nuggets of gold that you can apply to your own life, so you can experience similar results, quickly and profoundly.

Jenny is inspired by her Aunt Sue to choose the thoughts, emotions and habits that empower her to regain her energy and focus, so she can live with renewed passion and purpose. In other words, she learns to empower herself to achieve what we all desire and deserve: "Unstoppable Health."

So what exactly is "Unstoppable Health"? As I pondered the various words and phrases available to describe what I personally desire and what keeps me true to the habits that provide me the energy, joy and success I crave (and experience on a daily basis), many came to mind: Vibrant Health, Optimum Health, Radiant Health, Ideal Health – and more.

I chose "Unstoppable Health" because it encompasses all of those above and more. It brings into awareness that indeed, there *are* forces in the world that may try to "get in the way" of the habits required for feeling great all the time, and those need to be reckoned with.

So how do you do that? How do you deal with the forces that can sabotage your efforts to live better? You become connected and committed to your goals.

For me, I'm SO deeply connected and committed to what I want most, that when I come to a fork in the road - the daily choices that could tempt me away from my committed path - all I need to ask myself is "Which of the choices here keeps me aligned with my highest values and goals?" And the choice becomes obvious.

You see, Unstoppable Health is about knowing how to best nourish your body, mind and spirit. It's about creating habits that give you energy, clarity and joy. It's about not allowing obstacles to keep you from your deepest desires. It's about taking responsibility and surrounding yourself with others on the same path, and learning from mentors and teachers who've been there before.

Unstoppable Health requires daily practice and commitment.

Unstoppable Health requires shedding some old and comfortable habits, and donning new ones that free you to achieve the feelings and situations you most desire.

Unstoppable Health IS within reach. It's yours for the taking, IF you're willing to do the work.

Now, some people claim that "doing the work" required to achieve Unstoppable Health is "hard."

If you feel this way, too, I invite you to dive a little deeper into the concept of "hard."

Let's play a game.

Read through the choices below and **choose one or more of the situations that feel easier** than eating delicious whole fresh foods, establishing fun movement breaks each day, and letting go of limiting beliefs that hold you back.

1. Choosing to continue with the beliefs, thoughts and habits you inherited from your family and feeling run-down, stuck in a job you don't find fulfilling, and living in a body that causes you pain, discomfort, embarrassment or more.

2. Dealing with a chronic disease like diabetes, heart disease or autoimmunity, and all the possible interventions that western medicine offers, like open heart surgery, daily injections, and medications that simply manage the symptoms while the actual problem gets worse.

3. Missing out on key events in your life like weddings, graduations, special vacations, nights out with friends, and various hobbies, because you're too tired or sick to participate.

Seems pretty obvious which of the scenarios above would be truly "hard," right?

I urge you to redefine what "hard" really means to you. Often times, the reason you feel something is difficult is because you have no support, and you're confused about what to actually do to improve your health.

In this book, I'll introduce you to concepts and lifestyle changes that lead to Unstoppable Health. If you're already on the path to Unstoppable Health, that's great! Know that there's still much to learn, and keep reading to learn new strategies, and to figure out how to make sense of a lot of the conflicting health information available over the internet. Even better: get ready to adopt strategies that are personalized to *you*, so you increase your chances of success even more.

You'll also receive the same message several times as you read: it is so important to avoid making this journey on your own. Community is very important, and I will also share resources to help you get the support you need.

A quick side note about community – it's been scientifically proven that being a member of a community raises a person's level of a hormone called Oxytocin, which is the hormone of connection. Oxytocin engenders a feeling of safety, trust and love, and it's an important hormone if you desire to feel love, connection and joy – and we all have that deep yearning, don't we?

Throughout the book, I'll share my characters' recipes, activities, insights and ways they overcame their challenges. I've even created a special web-page where you can download the recipes and action steps you can implement to overcome your own challenges, and create Unstoppable Health for yourself. www.UnstoppableHealthResources.com

At the end of the book, there are additional resources to help you determine "where to go next," so that you can implement what you learn into your life.

What I desire most for you, as you read this book, is that you become excited to try out the quick and easy dishes (to which you have free access) that Aunt Sue introduces to Jenny as a way of changing her relationship with food and, as a consequence of that, her life.

The concepts I teach in this book are part of an emerging branch of health care called Nutritional Endocrinology™, and it's the root of my work with a growing number of health practitioners, including doctors, nurses, physician's assistants, nutritionists, acupuncturists, health coaches, counselors, and others who are interested in working with their patients and clients to get to the root cause of their ailments, rather than simply suppressing their symptoms – and THAT is my greatest hope: for our current disease management health care system to be replaced by one that is focused on getting to the root cause, rather than slapping a Band-Aid on the symptoms.

In reading "Unstoppable Health," you'll learn the basic foundations of Nutritional Endocrinology™, so you can restore balance to your hormones, digestion, and other body parts, and lead a life of joy, energy and focus.

So let's start this journey together, right now!

Pour yourself a cup of herbal tea, find a quiet spot and immerse yourself in the story that is about to unfold.

This is the first chapter in your life of "Unstoppable Health" – enjoy!

CHAPTER 1

Rock Bottom

P rofessor Howell hovered like a storm cloud over Jenny's desk, his florid face contorted with rage, his dark eyes piercing her tear-filled gaze. "What a fiasco! I've never been so embarrassed in all my time here. It hardly makes me look good having twenty faculty members waiting around for a presentation that almost didn't happen. Why? Because my assistant apparently forgot to book the audio visual equipment."

Her boss was now leaning so close that Jenny could smell the coffee on his breath. "I'm really tired of this, Jenny. You're totally unreliable and, frankly, I don't know what more I can do to get you to focus on your job so that I can do *mine*."

In the five years that Jenny had worked for the head of the university's Psychology Department, she'd never seen Professor Howell as furious as he was at that moment. She instinctively reached for the red stress ball that had become her much-needed crutch for moments like this. Once again, Jenny knew she had failed to demonstrate that she really was the efficient executive assistant she had once been. As she nervously contorted the rubber between her fingers in an unsuccessful attempt to control her rising panic, Jenny closed her eyes, desperately searching for a reason (any reason!) why the current "fiasco" really wasn't her fault.

Opening her eyes, Jenny immediately spotted the sticky note she had written to remind herself to book the necessary equipment for her boss' quarterly faculty meeting. It had become partially obscured by all the other reminders that were littering her computer screen.

Jenny felt the blood drain from her face, and her hands began to tremble. There was no way to wriggle out of this one; she was squarely, totally at fault.

It wasn't as if they hadn't been over this project several times in the past month: planning the stage layout, the equipment setup, the special speaker arrangement so Professor Howell could dominate the proceedings the way he preferred. To her boss, image was everything! Sure, he could have delivered the material largely without the use of any technology at all, but by utilizing all the new, state-of-the-art audio-visual equipment the department had just invested in, he could make himself look superior to those faculty members who could barely turn on their computers without assistance.

"Oh, no," Jenny mumbled under her breath. "I can't believe I forgot to do this."

Professor Howell took a deep breath and spoke slowly and deliberately, signaling his characteristic attempt at controlling his temper. "Jenny, what on earth is going on with you?" he asked.

There was an unnatural silence throughout the rest of the department. Given the open office layout, Jenny was acutely aware that all her co-workers were listening in to the conversation. She flushed with embarrassment, gripping the stress ball even more tightly.

Despite the deluge of thoughts going on in her mind, Jenny opened her mouth and croaked a timid: "I'm sorry. I guess I got so busy, I forgot, and my note ..." Her voice trailed off as she glanced up at Professor Howell's irate face. He was in no mood for excuses.

Own up to it. Tell him you take full responsibility, and ask what you can do to make up for it, Jenny's inner voice coached. "I'm so sorry, Professor Howell," she repeated, trying to meet his gaze with a confidence she didn't feel. "I know how important this meeting was and I blew it. It's all my fault. I accept that. Please tell me what I can do to make it right."

"How can you make something right that's already wrong? I looked like a complete fool up there," spat Professor Howell, shaking his head and throwing his arms up in the air. "Everyone had to sit around, twiddling their thumbs while we waited for facilities to bring in the equipment you promised to organize weeks ago. Really, I'm at a loss. Make it right? How?! Do tell, Jenny!"

Jenny looked down at the floor like a chided child. She so desperately wanted the day to be over.

But Professor Howell wasn't quite finished with her yet.

"This cannot happen again, Jenny. Do you understand? There have been far too many of these mix-ups with you lately and for the life of me, I can't understand why." Her boss sighed deeply. "When you started working for me five years ago, you were always so full of ideas, so energetic and ambitious. And it wasn't all that long ago that you asked if you could take on more responsibility. I was happy to accommodate you. But not now, not after this. Who in their right mind would give a person higher-level work to do, when she can't even handle the basic stuff adequately?"

"Professor Howell, I'm mortified by what's happened. Truly I am," Jenny blurted. "I realize how embarrassing this must have been for you. I know I need to improve my time-management skills. I'll do everything I can to bring those up to speed right away."

"Really?" Professor Howell responded skeptically. "I thought you were going to sign up for the productivity and time management seminar that Human Resources is sponsoring next week. Seems to me like you've even forgotten you'd committed yourself to that!"

Jenny looked down, feeling nauseous as she slumped even further into her chair. He was right; she'd forgotten to register for the course.

Professor Howell shook his head and shrugged. "You know something, Jenny? You can go and take that time-management course, but I don't think it's the answer. Seems to me you've lost all interest in this job, in working for me and this department. I don't know what caused that and frankly I don't care. I just need you to get your act together quickly, otherwise you and I will be sitting down very soon to discuss your future here." With that, Professor Howell turned his back and marched off in the direction of his office. Within seconds, she heard the slamming of a door.

The entire floor was now as silent as a grave. As the head of the department, Professor Howell's loud and public admonishment would no doubt be a source of office gossip for days. Jenny tried not to focus on that, realizing that it was the least of her problems.

She immediately went into a frenzy of activity, reaching for a lined pad on which to make a list of activities for Monday morning. At the top of that list was signing up for the time-management course. Maybe they could teach her a system for keeping track of all her to-dos that would work better than sticking dozens of Post-It notes on her computer screen and desk. Jenny knew something had to change. She also knew the problem was deeper than simply learning some new organizational strategies.

The trouble was, Jenny felt like her whole life needed a massive overhaul, but she was overwhelmed and clueless as to where to begin.

Still deep in thought, Jenny was startled when her cell phone vibrated, reminding her to lock her desk before heading home for the weekend. With a sigh of relief, she realized she could now go home and shut out the rest of the world, at least for the next two days.

"You ok, Jen?" It was Doris, the office manager, who had rushed to her side as Jenny quickly walked passed her co-worker's cubicle. Jenny murmured that she was fine as she picked up her pace. Reaching the exit, she felt the warm breeze envelop her face and, stepping out into the sunshine, she allowed the flood gates to open. She cried all the way to her car and during the entire long drive home.

* * *

Unlocking the door to her apartment, Jenny could hear her phone ringing. One. Two, Three. Four. Five. After five rings, it went to voicemail. She absentmindedly dropped her purse inside the door, kicked off her shoes, and flopped down on the couch, so tired that she couldn't even be bothered to go through her usual ritual of changing out of her office clothes.

"What on earth is happening to me?" she asked herself, and waited, as if expecting some new insight to pop into her head. But all she heard was the replay of Professor Howell's voice telling her she was stupid, inefficient, disorganized, and if she wasn't careful, soon to be out of a job. In an attempt to stop the mental movie playing over and over in her head, Jenny reached for the remote control and clicked on the TV.

Flicking through the channels, trying to find something other than car and pharmaceutical drug commercials, Jenny jolted to a stop as she came across the image of a beautiful woman around her own age – late thirties - who was perched atop a sleek racing bike, her long slender legs topped with dark blue Spandex shorts. Smiling directly at the camera to reveal her unusually white teeth, looking energized and joyous, the woman began talking about her plans to cycle across the country to raise money for children affected by recent natural disasters in her state.

"When did I stop wanting to be like her?," Jenny wondered, looking disgustedly at her overweight body, feeling drained of energy as she lay curled up on the couch, stripped of ambition, hope and purpose. "I always thought I would do something important with my life." Feeling tortured (rather than inspired) by the image of this slim, beautiful person who was on a mission to do something meaningful, Jenny switched off the TV set and threw down the remote.

"Where's my life going?" she asked out loud, surprised by the bitterness in her voice. Jenny glanced over at the stack of exercise videos, the weights, the yoga mat and other paraphernalia that was lying on the other side of the room, neatly organized, ready for action, none of which had been touched in months.

"I'm stuck in a dead-end job with a boss who hates me, I'm carrying 20 pounds more than I was this time last year, and I barely have the energy to get myself off this couch to make dinner."

The thought of a meal made Jenny realize how ravenous she was. Easing herself off the couch, she headed to the kitchen and opened the refrigerator door.

The first thing that caught her eye was a half-empty, uncovered carton of yogurt, complete with the spoon she had used to eat it sticking out of the top. Reaching in, Jenny was almost to the point of licking the spoon when she caught a sour whiff. She sighed deeply as she tossed the whole thing, including the silverware, into the trash. Returning to the fridge, Jenny realized there was nothing edible to be found. It was to be a Diet Coke dinner, tonight. In disgust, she slammed the refrigerator door closed with the sole of her foot.

That's when she caught a glimpse of her shopping list sticky note on the fridge door. She'd intended to go to the grocery store on her way home from work, but had forgotten to take the reminder note. She certainly wasn't in the mood now, but what she wouldn't give for a slice of chocolate cake or a carton full of ice cream!

As she headed toward the pantry, Jenny realized she was unlikely to find anything worth eating in there, either. She scanned the shelves and sure enough, she was right; she reached for a bag of potato chips, then headed back to the living room and flopped down on the couch. *Another chips and Coke night - what a feast*, Jenny scolded herself. *Still, at least this will fill me up for now. I'll go shopping tomorrow*, she decided, as she popped open the can of soda and ripped the bag of chips with her teeth.

Jenny was startled out of her thoughts by the shrill ring of her cell phone. Picking it up, she glanced at the screen before answering. It was her best friend, Joy, the one person she'd been able to count on since high school. Jenny picked up the phone, and feigning cheerfulness, said, "Hey there, Joy, how are you?"

"Hi. Where are you? I hit quite a bit of traffic and was wondering if that's what's holding you up."

"What do you mean traffic?" said Jenny. "I'm here at home."

There followed what felt to Jenny like a very long pause before Joy responded. Jenny knew when that happened, her friend was irritated.

When Joy did speak, it was slow and deliberate: "You ... were supposed to ... meet me at Forrest Park. Remember? Hiking? The fundraiser?"

Another long pause.

"Jenny, for goodness sake, I watched you write this down on your calendar!"

Jenny immediately walked back to the kitchen and looked at the calendar; she didn't remember making any such plans. She turned over the pages until she reached the correct month, and there it was, in bold letters: "Joy. Forrest Park, 6:00 pm hike & meet."

Jenny stood, open-mouthed and horrified at her failing memory. She was only 37 years old. What in the world was going on? Surely this wasn't a good sign!

"You still there?" Jenny stammered. "I'm so sorry, Joy, I completely forgot. You won't believe this, but I don't even have the right month showing. I just didn't see that we had plans tonight."

"Please don't make this out as if it's a rare occurrence, Jenny. Let's be honest, I can count five times in the past few weeks that we've made plans and you've either cancelled at the last minute, or were a no-show for whatever reason: you're too tired, too sick, or not in the mood. What the hell is up with you? If you don't want to see or do things with me, then at least have the guts to say so!"

Jenny's first attempt to speak sounded like a strangled gasp. She took a deep breath, and blurted out, "It's just not fair. People get sick, Joy. Aren't you ever too tired to go out?

It happens to everyone." As she spoke those words, she felt increasingly worse at having let her friend down. "Look, I just had a day from hell at work. My boss went off the deep end in front of everyone. Now you're yelling at me for messing up ..."

"Jenny, I gotta go," Joy interrupted. "Everyone's waiting for me. I'm sorry you had a bad day. Maybe it's just as well you're not here, if you're in a mood. On the other hand, it probably would have helped you to feel better. I'll call you over the weekend. Or you call me. Whatever." Jenny whispered goodbye as the line disconnected.

She was alone again with only her thoughts for company - not much of a way to spend Friday evening.

She glanced back at the calendar, and flipped through the previous three months. Joy was right; Jenny had cancelled several plans with her, feeling too tired, having forgotten, or because she'd double-booked herself several times.

"What *is* going on with me?" Jenny asked herself. "Why am I always so tired? What's with all this memory loss?"

As she dragged herself back to the living room, and slumped down onto the couch, Jenny acknowledged again how exhausted she felt. She grabbed a handful of chips, washed them down with a big gulp of Coke, and headed toward the bedroom, feeling the best thing she could do was go to bed early and hope everything would look better in the morning.

Her laptop lay on the unmade bed, the screen still open. Jenny decided to check her email before turning in.

As she scrolled through the usual spam and newsletters that filled her Inbox, one email address caught her eye ... Susan Phillips. The name was familiar, but Jenny couldn't place it immediately. It certainly wasn't one of her usual email correspondents.

Then it hit her. The email was from her mother's sister, Aunt Sue. Jenny hadn't heard from her aunt in years. Thinking that it must be important, Jenny clicked on the email and began reading:

Hi Jenny,

Surprise! I know it's been ages since we last communicated, but I'm coming to your neck of the woods! Got a lot going on in the next few weeks: a conference, a race, and a few client meetings. Will be in your city for almost a month and am hoping you might take some time off for play. Also, if it's not too much of an imposition, I thought it might be fun to stay at your place. Just let me know if that would work ... I promise not to shake up your world too much - LOL. Attached is my flight itinerary and a brief schedule of events. So looking forward to catching up on all your news!

Much love,

Aunt Sue

Jenny felt like crying again, but the well was dry. She slammed the laptop lid shut; she'd respond in the morning when she felt a little calmer. *Fun? She's got to be joking. I can barely keep my act together by myself. The last thing I need right now is a house guest.*

Feeling totally exhausted, Jenny turned off the bedroom light and lay there, listening to her breath and the continual chatter in her brain. She never went to bed *this* early, yet she didn't have the energy or heart to do anything else. Habitually, she reached over to the bottle of melatonin tablets lying on the bedside cabinet, removed two and washed them down with a gulp of flat, warm soda left over from the night before.

Jenny reviewed the day; it was not one of her better ones. Her job was on the line, her memory seemed to be on permanent vacation, and she'd ticked off her longest and dearest friend. And if that wasn't enough, she now had an elderly relative wanting to be her houseguest for almost a month.

It took several hours before Jenny's mind quieted down enough for her to get some fitful sleep.

CHAPTER 2

Time for Change

I can't believe she's planning to stay a whole month," complained Jenny, slumping further into her friend Patty's sofa during their customary Saturday get-together.

"Can't you just say you're busy?" asked Patty, gulping a Diet Coke. "I'll be your alibi, if you like. After all, what are best friends for?" She reached into the bag of chips that was lying between them on the coffee table, grabbed a handful, and after smearing each one liberally with sour cream dip, continued her objection to Jenny's aunt's visit, regardless of the fact that the two had never met.

Holding the chip in midair, Patty glared at Jenny, pursed her lips and said, "The nerve of the woman! After all, a whole month? You won't have any privacy. What if she expects you to clean up after her? And it sounds like she thinks you're just going to drop everything to entertain her. Really, Jenny, do you need that extra stress? After what's just happened with your boss and Joy being on your case? Remember when that cousin of mine was here from California? She only stayed a week, but it drove me half crazy. The longest week of my life, I swear. Okay, girlfriend, we're just going to have to figure out how to get you out of it."

Jenny grimaced, not wishing to contradict her friend. Having slept on the idea, she woke actually looking forward to Aunt Sue's visit. After all, something needed to change in her life. Even if she wasn't thrilled at the prospect of entertaining a houseguest for a whole month, it *would* shake up her humdrum existence. And it would be nice to have the company.

"Yeah, it's a drag," said Jenny, trying to maintain the connection with her friend. "But I can't just lie. She's family and we have to be there for one other. It wouldn't be right to make Aunt Sue stay in a hotel for all that time when I've got a perfectly good guest room she can use. My parents would be really ticked off at me if they found out, which they would. Look, she's coming in two weeks and I'm just going to have to figure out how to survive it. Really, it won't be that bad."

Jenny looked wistfully across her friend's patio, beyond the chain link fence to the walking trails where a young woman was jogging past with her dog. She recalled a time not too long ago when she used to jog on those trails, the breeze warm and fresh across her sweaty brow, invigorated by the effort as she pushed herself harder and harder against the steep hills in the Preserve. Joy would often join her, and they'd push each other to achieve even further distances.

"Hey, why don't we go outside to sit?" Jenny asked her friend, as she got up from the sofa and began walking toward the patio door. "After all, it's a beautiful day. Maybe being out in the sun will cheer me up a bit."

"Do we have to? I'm comfortable where I am," Patty replied, her large body barely stirring from her curled position on the sofa. "Besides, the sun is so bright and the kids playing down below are so noisy and ..." Her voice trailed off as Patty struggled to sit up, having noticed that Jenny had already opened the door, letting in a light breeze.

"Oh, all right, if you really want to," Patty sighed.

Jenny noticed the irritated look on her friend's face, but stood defiantly for several minutes, watching Patty as she wriggled and writhed to free her overweight frame from the comfortable grasp of the voluminous couch cushions.

Jenny turned back toward the coffee table, grabbed the bag of chips they'd been snacking on and headed outside. As she plopped herself down on a large cushioned chair, she breathed an audible sigh. A warm breeze softly blew her shoulder length blonde hair forward into her face. Below them a group of children were playing, laughing and running gleefully. A few buds had already begun to bloom in the flowerbeds that had been dug between the apartment complex and the walking path. As she took a deep breath, Jenny could sense the fragrance of newly cut grass, and she smiled slightly.

"I should use the next two weeks to get serious about losing some weight. The last time Aunt Sue saw me, I was at least 30 pounds lighter." Jenny paused in recollection before continuing. "I still have the dress I wore that day, at my sister's wedding. Funny, I spotted it in the closet this morning. It's hanging with all the other great clothes I used to wear, before ..." Jenny's voice trailed off. She suddenly felt a deep sense of sadness, longing, and frustration as she wistfully recalled happier times. Jenny bit her lip and clasped her hands tightly. "I felt great whenever I wore that dress. It really showed off the curves I used to have, and turned a lot of heads."

"Oh Jenny, get over it! You look great the way you are. You're not going to fit into those clothes again. You've been trying - and not very successfully I might add - for the past three years. Give them away. Don't torture yourself by looking at them. I can't understand why you let this bother you so much. It's only natural to get bigger as we age. Being voluptuous doesn't bother me, and it shouldn't bother you either."

"I was wearing that dress the first time I met Tom," Jenny continued, ignoring Patty's protests. "He couldn't take his eyes off me. I want that again, Patty. I want to ..."

Patty interrupted Jenny mid-sentence. "Is that what this is all about Jenny? Men? Like we haven't had enough trouble with them over the years? I don't think you want me to remind you how it turned out with Tom."

Patty's words stung Jenny deeply. She started to protest, but stopped herself. They'd covered this topic many times before and it was always the same. They weren't overweight; they were "voluptuous." They weren't lonely, they were "self-sufficient." They weren't unfulfilled; they were just being practical. Patty's view of the world seemed to be so different from Jenny's, but she no longer had the energy to argue. And anyhow, maybe Patty was right. Jenny didn't know what was true for her anymore.

"I need to go home now," Jenny said suddenly as she stood up and began gathering her things.

"What d'you mean, 'go home'? It's still early and we were going to watch a movie together. I already took out the frozen pizzas to heat up for dinner."

"I just remembered I've laundry to do, and grocery shopping," Jenny lied. "I'll call you later." Jenny was through the front door before Patty could heave herself up out of the chair. She heard her friend call her name as the door slammed shut behind her.

CHAPTER 3

A New Beginning

It had been ten years since Jenny had seen her Aunt Sue, and without a recent picture to go by, Jenny hoped the internal picture she had of her mother's 64-year old sister was still accurate. Standing in the airport, watching streams of weary passengers trudge into the main concourse, Jenny scrutinized every gray-haired woman she saw. She checked her watch.

Did I get the time wrong?, she wondered as the last stragglers strolled through the gate. *Maybe she stopped at the bathroom,* Jenny thought. Then she jumped, startled by a gentle tap on her shoulder.

"Jenny?"

The younger woman turned, and let out a gasp, "Aunt Sue?"

A beautiful dark-haired woman stood before her, looking not a day older than in her late forties. She set down her carry-on bag and reached out to hug Jenny. The older woman's energy, despite having just completed a full day's journey, was palpable.

"It's so wonderful to see you again, my dear," exclaimed Sue, holding her niece at arm's length and looking her up and down. "I can't believe we let it go so long before re-connecting. We're going to need almost a month together just to catch up on the news! I can't wait to hear everything about your life. I only hope it's treating you as well as mine is me!"

Jenny just stood there, knowing she must look very much like a goldfish, the way her mouth opened and closed. A million thoughts ran through her mind, but she had no idea where to start. Sue appeared not to have aged *at all* over the previous ten years. If anything, she actually seemed more vibrant, trim and healthy than how Jenny remembered her; she practically glowed!

The two women linked arms and began walking toward the luggage carousels. "I can't believe how amazing you look," Jenny said. "There I was, checking out all the grandmotherly types and here you are, looking so incredibly glamorous and fit! You're going to have to let me into your secret. Lord knows, I need it."

"You're a sweetheart for saying so, my dear," said Sue. "It's true; I do have a few travel rituals I use to keep me fresh while I fly. Remind me to share them with you later."

Sue had obviously misunderstood Jenny's remark. She didn't want to know how her aunt managed to look so rested after a long flight. She wanted to know how Sue looked so young - close to her own age, in fact, despite the 27-year age gap.

"About my luggage," Sue laughed as they stood by the carousel, eyeing the bags and boxes that were strewn along the moving conveyer belt. "I hope your car has a good sized trunk."

Jenny blushed. She had meant to clean out her car before Sue's visit and suddenly realized that was another thing on her to-do list that was still pending.

Sue moved toward a huge suitcase, her hand outstretched to grab the handle. Jenny instinctively tried to take over. "Let me get that for you," she said.

"No worries, honey, I have it," said Sue, hoisting the suitcase off the conveyer belt and onto a luggage cart with ease.

As Jenny watched her aunt claim two other sizeable bags, she was in awe of the older woman's strength and agility. "Well, you certainly seem to have kept yourself fit," said Jenny.

Sue beamed. "Actually, I feel quite invigorated. It's so exciting to visit new places, don't you find? And being with you is cause for celebration!"

Jenny pushed the trolley toward the exit that would take them to the parking lot where she had left her midsize vehicle.

"Would you like to grab a bite to eat?" Jenny asked, as they passed the food court. "I bet you're really hungry after your travels. I can't imagine they gave you much on the flight."

"I brought some fruit and travel snacks to munch on the plane, so I'm doing just fine, really," said Sue.

"But, yes, dinner at your house sounds fantastic! Here's what I'm thinking: I looked online and saw you have several health food stores and supermarkets with organic sections that we could stop off at on the way. Let's drop by one of those and get what we need to prepare a light supper. How does that sound?"

Sue mentioned the names of several stores that Jenny had not yet visited. Her friend Joy often shopped at these stores, and they had even made plans to go to them together sometime.

Jenny laughed at Sue's excited suggestion of conjuring up a meal together, and said "I can't think of the last time I made anything but toast in my kitchen! But I have to admit, that sounds fun." Jenny found herself instinctively responding to her aunt's energy and enthusiasm, and noticed that she had doubled her normal walking pace in order to keep up, as they walked to Jenny's car.

Opening the trunk, the two women peered incredulously from it to the mountain of luggage that Sue had brought with her. Jenny silently cursed herself for not having emptied her vehicle of its typical detritus - books she still had to take back to the library, a gym bag with clothing that had not seen the light of day for many months, and some clothes she no longer fit in that she had finally decided to take to the Goodwill, but had never gotten around to actually dropping off.

Suddenly a man appeared, as if out of nowhere, and said, "Perhaps I can help you?" After an appreciative nod from Sue, he got to work helping to move Jenny's belongings into the back seat, to create more room in the trunk.

"That should do it," the man said after fitting in the final piece of jigsaw puzzle luggage. He turned directly to face Sue, who smiled at him warmly, her beautiful face slightly tinged with pink.

"Thank you so much. You're quite the knight in shining armor," she said.

The man, who Jenny thought resembled Tom Selleck, reached out to shake her aunt's hand and said with obvious sincerity, "It's been a pleasure meeting you." He paused a little longer than normal, seeming reluctant to walk away.

"Off we go, then," said Sue, winking at Jenny who had never experienced anything like what had just happened, before.

"That man was flirting with you," said Jenny, as she started up the engine and eased her car into the parking garage's exit lane. She felt a pang of envy as her aunt - over a quarter of a century older - explained that this happened to her all the time. "Isn't it *wonderful,* being a woman?" Jenny didn't reply. She couldn't remember the last time she had felt that way; it certainly hadn't been any time recently.

After driving several miles in silence, Sue turned to acknowledge the back seat bulging with Jenny's things, and laughed. "Let's just pick up a few goodies at the store. We can do a bigger shopping trip tomorrow when we've a bit more room."

At the grocery store, Sue headed determinedly for the produce aisle. Jenny followed behind.

"What kind of greens would you prefer in your salad, Jenny? There's romaine, spring mix, green leaf. Then there's arugula, or spinach ... that can be a tasty combination too."

Jenny had never thought about what kind of lettuce she preferred. In fact, she had no idea that there even were so many choices. "I typically just get a head of iceberg," Jenny said.

"Then let me welcome to the wonderful world of green goodies," smiled Sue. "Let's get a few varieties. I think you'll find these have a bit more character than what you're used to." Sue picked up several containers with names that Jenny was not familiar with and began pushing the cart further into the produce section.

Sue strode down the aisles like a woman "on a mission," placing tomatoes, kale, scallions, and cilantro into the cart. Jenny had never visited this particular store, and certainly didn't tend to spend much time in the produce section; she was amazed at the variety of vegetables Aunt Sue was choosing. After selecting carrots, celery, red bell peppers and avocados, her aunt turned to Jenny and asked, "Any idea where the Asian section is? I'd like to pick up some sea vegetables."

"Sea vegetables? What are they? I don't think I've ever had sea vegetables."

"Then you're in for a treat, my dear. I'm going to make you my **sesame ginger sea salad**. You'll love it!"

Jenny thought that eating vegetables grown in sea water sounded downright weird, but she decided to trust that her aunt knew what she was doing.

"Jenny, do you have a water filter in your apartment? Or should we buy some bottled water?"

"There's a filter on the refrigerator but it's glowing red and obviously needs changing. Sorry, I haven't gotten around to it. The tap water tastes just fine, though. I don't notice a difference except for the temperature. I usually fill up some of those plastic bottles with tap water and keep them cold."

"How about we buy a bottle of Mountain Spring water?" said Aunt Sue. "I haven't drank tap water ever since I found out about all the chemicals they use to purify it. Did you know that the chlorine in tap water can harm your thyroid gland? And they've even found traces of prescription drugs in tap water," Sue said matter-of-factly as she scanned the overhead signs.

Jenny held onto the shopping cart in order to keep up. "You know, I figured water is water, and all this hype about buying it in bottles was just a money-making scheme. In any case, I've heard that the plastic that bottled water comes in introduces toxins that are worse than just drinking the water out of the tap."

Sue cocked her head to one side. "Some of that's true, Jenny," she said after a brief pause. "When plastics are heated, like when you leave a plastic water bottle in the car on a hot day, it accelerates the breakdown of chemicals known as xeno-estrogens, and they get into the water."

The two women were now walking down the beverage aisle. Sue continued, "Xeno-estrogens can certainly interfere with your hormone balance and cause all sorts of unpleasant side effects. That's why I try to buy my water in glass containers - eliminating those kinds of risks. Whenever I take water with me in the car, I use either glass or stainless steel bottles."

Jenny was amazed. Sue was like a walking health encyclopedia. "How come you know so much about water?"

Sue giggled. "Actually, it's part of my work. My company distributes water filters and, as one of their sales and marketing reps, I've been to many trainings and had to do a lot of research. My customers want to feel confident that I know what I'm talking about, as opposed to just trying to sell them stuff. I'd actually thought about bringing one of our top-of-the-line filters with me," Sue continued, "but I wanted to wait and see what you had first. We'll take a look at your apartment and I'll order you a filter for your kitchen and your shower."

Jenny stared in amazement. *A shower filter? Why would I need that?* she wondered, but didn't want to seem even more ignorant than she had appeared about bottled water. Her brain was already starting to pound from all she'd learned from Sue so far. Besides, Jenny was hungry; the sooner they finished shopping and got home, the sooner she could eat.

At the checkout counter, Sue struck up a friendly conversation with the cashier, who asked what she was planning to do with so many vegetables, fruits, and green food. Sue laughed warmly, saying, "Oh, I'm going to make my niece here a meal to remember."

* * *

With the last of the luggage and groceries now in Jenny's small apartment, Aunt Sue began washing her hands in the kitchen sink.

"Let's get started with dinner right away, Jenny, so we don't eat too late," she said. "I like to finish eating at least a few hours before bedtime, so I can have a more restful sleep."

"What does the time you eat have to do with how restful your sleep is?" Jenny asked.

Sue searched through Jenny's kitchen drawers until she found a sharp knife, and then began rummaging through the shopping bags, pulling out various packages and setting them on the counter.

"Whenever you move, breathe, think or get stressed-out, your body generates waste products and toxins. These build up throughout the day, making you feel tired later." Aunt Sue offered, continuing to organize the groceries. "Think of sleep as the time that your body's cleanup crew goes to work, eliminating those wastes, so you feel refreshed in the morning. If you eat right before bed, you spend several hours digesting your food, and that all-important clean-up just doesn't happen. That's why you feel tired in the morning, especially after a big, heavy meal the night before. If I have to eat late for whatever reason, such as when I'm traveling or meeting clients for business dinners, I'll always choose lighter, easy-to-digest foods."

"Oh, you mean like a sandwich instead of a full meal? I do that sometimes," Jenny responded.

Sue threw back her head and laughed, then squeezed Jenny's arm affectionately. "Well, not exactly, Jenny, but you have the right idea. Sandwiches are smaller than a full course meal, but they're still pretty difficult to digest. Think of all that bread, let alone the meat and mayonnaise that folks put in a typical sandwich. By lighter, more easily digested foods, I'm talking about things like fresh fruits, salads and smoothies."

"Ah, diet food! "Jenny replied, thinking that she was beginning to catch on.

"Yes, fresh fruits and veggies are usually considered diet foods because they're loaded with nutrition and low in calories," said Sue, adding, "Jenny, I think I have everything I need for the moment. Why don't you go ahead and unpack the rest of this and put it in your refrigerator? It's not a good idea to have these fresh foods sitting out for too long."

As she followed her aunt's instruction, Jenny was struck by how much green food was in the bags. She couldn't resist pointing out that she didn't even have that much green on her lawn.

"Just wait until you taste how delicious this food is," replied Aunt Sue. "Don't worry; I'm not trying to turn you into a rabbit."

Jenny grimaced, aware of the rumbling noises coming from her empty stomach, and she resisted the urge to dive into the pantry and raid the cookie jar. She wasn't convinced that salad stuff was going to make her feel satisfied, and she envisioned herself tip-toeing into the kitchen for a midnight snack.

"Do you have your blender handy, darling? I know you're hungry and I'd like to make us a quick energy drink before we get started," said Sue casually, as if she had read Jenny's mind.

Jenny had to think for several minutes. *Where was the blender?* It had been at least a year and a half since she had last used it ... for the margarita party she and Joy had hosted when friends of theirs had become engaged.

After rummaging around in several cupboards and pulling out pans and other kitchen gadgets that were still in their boxes, unused, Jenny found the blender.

"Seems you've had this for a while," said Sue, not un-kindly. "It's a bit small and not very powerful, but it'll do for now. Let's be sure to add a blender to our list for our next shopping trip. That'll be my treat in exchange for being here a whole month. Better yet, I should order you a Vitamix, my favorite kitchen appliance. I must admit, I'm addicted to my smoothies and dips, and having a Vitamix to work with while I'm here will make me very happy!"

Jenny watched Sue as she threw into the blender a small container of precut pineapple and mango chunks, a splash of freshly squeezed organic lime juice, a half inch piece of ginger, and the entire contents of a container of prewashed baby spinach.

Sue measured out a cup of the spring water from the glass bottles they'd bought, added a handful of ice cubes and ran the blender until the concoction was smooth, creamy and bright green.

She divided up the drink, pouring it into two large wine glasses, and handed one to Jenny

Jenny stared at the green concoction, trying to mask any looks that would reveal what was running through her head - that something that looked so disgusting had to taste that way too. She sniffed it surreptitiously. It smelled more tropical than its color suggested it would.

Sue held up her glass and clinked it against Jenny's, saying, "Cheers ... here's to a fabulous visit." Bringing the glass up to her mouth, Sue took a long slow swallow.

Jenny stared at her own glass gingerly. She didn't want to appear rude, but wondered how she was going to stomach drinking something that looked like liquidized grass clippings.

Aunt Sue moved closer to her niece and whispered conspiratorially: "It's hard to get over the color, isn't it? I remember when I was offered my very first green smoothie, I was horrified at the prospect. After all, we're not used to drinking green things. It seems so alien to us, like downing blended lawn pulp."

Jenny laughed at her aunt's empathetic assessment of her thoughts at that moment.

"Auntie, you just nailed it. You're right, I've never drank anything green before. It's hard not to think it's going to taste gross. Actually, what does it taste like?"

Aunt Sue smiled gently. "Much like a tropical fruit drink. Go ahead, try it and see. You'll like it, I promise. After all, you've already said you like mango and pineapple. Go on, be brave. Let me know what you think."

Jenny continued to hesitate, thinking that if she drank it with her eyes closed she could get past the vivid grassy color. She took a deep breath instead, lifted the glass to her lips and sipped tentatively - first a tiny drop, then a little more, then a full mouthful.

Jenny looked across at her aunt, who was eyeing her expectantly.

"It's really good, "Jenny said, as if not believing her own taste buds. "It tastes really sweet, quite delicious actually - no green taste at all. It's quite bizarre; I'd never have thought something that looks like this could taste so good. Whatever possessed you to blend up such an unusual concoction in the first place?" Jenny asked.

Aunt Sue put her own drink down on the counter and moved over to hug her niece.

"Let's just say I'm always open to new experiences," Sue laughed. "And when someone told me that these drinks could increase my energy levels, I figured that since I still have a lot of life to live, it made sense to fuel my body this way. There's more where this came from. You'll get to try a lot of my concoctions before too long."

Sue turned back to the counter where she had assembled the ingredients for the main meal.

"Come on. Let's make dinner. I'm starving. Jenny, get your food processor out and we'll get started."

In her search for the blender, Jenny at least knew where this item was - still in the box she had received it in as a gift, some years earlier. She felt embarrassed that it had never been used.

"Never got round to working out what I needed this for," Jenny mumbled as if in apology.

Her aunt removed the processor from its packaging to inspect it. "How cute ... a mini food processor. It'll do for now. Tomorrow we'll get you a full-sized one. We're going to need it!"

Again, Jenny watched as Sue threw into the bowl a handful each of raw almonds and sunflower seeds, a scallion, a roughly chopped stalk of celery, a few spices and a dash of sea salt. After a few minutes of processing, the consistency resembled **Tuna Salad**. After tasting it herself and adding a little more celery, Sue inserted a fresh teaspoon, scooped up some of the concoction and handed it to Jenny to taste. "What do you think of this?"

Jenny was now feeling braver after the experience with the **Green Smoothie**. She took the proffered spoon and placed its contents in her mouth. "This is delicious. Can't wait to eat the whole thing," she said enthusiastically.

Jenny continued to watch curiously as Aunt Sue created her promised **Ginger Seaweed Salad**. She took a handful of what looked like black spaghetti, informing Jenny that its proper name was *arame*. Sue soaked the *arame* in a bowl of water for five minutes until it had swollen to three times its size. Then she chopped up garlic, ginger, basil and cilantro, shredded a couple of carrots, and added it to the *arame*. A few drops of sesame oil, a dash of flax oil, and a pinch of sea salt, and Sue pronounced the dish ready.

The whole dish had taken ten minutes to prepare, at most. With the smoothie as an appetizer and the dessert she'd quickly rustled up before they sat down for dinner, Sue had prepared a three-course meal for two in under an hour.

"Tell me again why this sea spaghetti stuff is good for me?" Jenny asked, as she savored a forkful.

"Sea vegetables are fabulous sources of nutrition, Jenny. They concentrate the minerals from the ocean and provide them to us in dense little packages. They are the best source of iodine, too, which is deficient in most soils. You need iodine for your thyroid gland, which helps boost your metabolism, which in turn helps maintain your ideal body weight. Plus, sea veggies are wonderful for helping rid your body of excess heavy metals and toxins."

Jenny couldn't believe how much she liked the food! Aunt Sue seemed to Jenny a magician, as she transformed the unfamiliar ingredients on the counter into delicious dishes, some of which resembled foods that Jenny had eaten before.

For dessert, they had **Chocolate Mousse**, whipped up in a matter of minutes using avocado, zucchini, organic chocolate powder, a pinch of vanilla and a natural, no-calorie sweetener which Aunt Sue had brought from home called Chinese Luo Han, also known as monk fruit. The thick, creamy sweet pudding tasted similar to what her mom used to make for Jenny when she was a child, although making whipped cream out of nuts and coconut seemed surrealistic.

"You're a wizard in the kitchen, Aunt Sue," said Jenny, realizing how pleasantly sated she felt. She felt no desire or need to raid the pantry for cookies any time soon.

"You ain't seen nothing yet," Sue said. "They say a change is as good as a rest. Are you up for some change in your life, Jenny?"

Jenny nodded, thinking to herself, *you have no idea!*

CHAPTER 4

Change is in the Air

Sunlight streamed into Jenny's bedroom. She glanced at the bedside clock, surprised to find that it was fifteen minutes *before* the alarm was set to go off. Jenny almost never woke up before her alarm, and certainly hadn't done so for years. She felt a surge of panic, as she heard someone moving around outside her bedroom door and automatically looked for something she could use in self-defense. Then she remembered, and she lay back against the warm pillows and smiled: it was Saturday, there was no need to get ready for work and, better still, the footsteps she heard were her wonderful aunt's!

Recalling the previous evening they'd enjoyed filled Jenny with anticipation – she wondered what her aunt had planned for breakfast! It had been a long time since she had focused on food with any sense of adventure or delight.

Jenny threw on a robe and opened the bedroom door just in time to hear the front door click shut. Rushing into the living room, Jenny caught a glimpse of her aunt through the glass door, looking slim and fit in spandex running shorts and a fitted tank top. *She looks amazing*, thought Jenny, as she suddenly came to the realization that none of the women she knew, with the exception of Joy, looked as sleek and athletic as her aunt, despite being a generation younger. Feeling a pang of disappointment at having missed her aunt, Jenny headed to the kitchen to make herself a cup of coffee.

A note from her aunt was the first thing she saw, propped up against the bowl of fruit:

Off for a run ... back in an hour. Smoothie for you in the fridge - keen to hear what you think of this one. We'll go shopping later. Love u. S.

Jenny smiled as she opened the refrigerator door to find a jar of what looked like blended houseplants. She remembered how surprisingly delicious the last green smoothie had tasted, and hoped that this one was going to be similarly palatable.

Pouring the green concoction into a wine glass, Jenny grabbed the morning newspaper as she made her way toward the patio door. Not used to being up so early on a Saturday morning, Jenny was immediately filled with a sense of peace at how beautiful this time of day could be, the only sounds being the morning calls of birds. After drinking the smoothie, Jenny felt no need to make coffee. With a spring in her step, she zipped through her Saturday morning rituals, and was pulling on her jeans when she heard the front door open.

Jenny rushed to the entry way to greet her aunt, who looked up in surprise.

"Well, hi there. You're up bright and early. Hope I didn't disturb you when I left the apartment. I figured I'd get out for a run before you got up."

"Not at all," said Jenny. "In fact, I saw you jog away. I know I said last night that I planned to sleep in, but I woke up feeling so great I figured I'd get dressed and grab some breakfast. Thanks for the smoothie, by the way. Totally delicious." Jenny hugged her aunt in appreciation before asking, "How was your run?"

"Great! I love going out just after the sun comes up. There's something about that peace and the light that sets me up for the rest of the day."

"So where did you go?" Jenny asked.

Her aunt told her about finding the jogging path that led to the nearby woods and how she had completed a lap around the lake.

"Have you done that recently?" Aunt Sue asked.

"Not for a long while," said Jenny. "My friend Joy and I used to do it at least a couple of times a week."

"Why did you stop?" Sue asked.

Jenny replied, "Oh, Joy got a new job and moved across town to be closer to her office. We planned to get together and do it on the weekends, but somehow I never got around to it. Unexpected things kept cropping up, you know?" Jenny was immediately struck by the realization that Joy had been so much more diligent at maintaining their friendship, planning all sorts of events that Jenny had canceled because she didn't have the energy. "Work keeps me pretty busy and exercise just kind of fell by the wayside."

"It's so much easier to stay committed when you're accountable to someone else, don't you find?" asked Sue. "How about you and me do this together every morning while I'm here? I know I'd enjoy the company."

Jenny looked aghast. "Thanks, but I don't think you'd want that. I'm so out of shape and tired all the time that I wouldn't keep up. I'd likely poop out after ten minutes!"

"Then we'll do ten minutes, and work up from there," said Sue. "It'll be fun! I can get things started for you, and then you can pick up with your friend Joy. That is, if you really want to."

"I do. Kind of," said Jenny unconvincingly. "To be honest, I've started and stopped more diet and exercise regimes than I dare count. Look at that pile of exercise videos," she added, pointing toward the television. "Most of them are still in the shrink wrap!"

Aunt Sue moved across the kitchen and put her arms around her niece, giving her a gentle squeeze. "You know, my dear, I have a feeling that once you get started again, and really commit to taking small steps every single day, you'll see your life change right before your very eyes. It'll be quite magical, I bet. Think about it. We can get started tomorrow!

I need to go take a shower and then we can talk about how the rest of the day is shaping up. Do you have anything already scheduled, that we need to work around?"

"Nope, I cleared my calendar to spend the day with you," Jenny said, blushing at the half-truth. In reality, the only thing she ever did on Saturdays was her laundry. She usually hung out with Patty, too, but Jenny had already informed her friend that since it was Aunt Sue's first day, she wouldn't be able to make their usual get-together.

Patty had been annoyed when Jenny had told her about this change of plans, saying, "Don't go turning your life around for her, Jenny. Let her fend for herself. She can't expect you to just drop your friends because she's here."

The truth was, Jenny had been looking for an excuse for a while to get out of her Saturday rut with Patty, especially now that the weather was becoming warmer. Unfortunately,

Patty was never interested in doing anything that didn't involve gossiping on her sofa, or pigging out as they watched movies together.

Jenny was still contemplating how boring and routine her life had become when Aunt Sue re-emerged, fresh from her shower, looking stunning in tight grey jeans and a sapphire blue T-shirt.

"I meant to tell you earlier," said Jenny. "I loved the drink you made me for breakfast. It kind of smelled like Pina Colada, so I pretended I was on a tropical island, with warm breezes blowing through my hair and that I was drinking a cocktail. Really, it was delicious. What was in it?"

"Let's see," Aunt Sue mused as she rummaged through Jenny's kitchen cupboards with a lined pad and pen in hand, making notes. "Remember the Thai coconut we bought last night, the one you said was shaped like a circus tent? I poked a hole in the top and poured the juice into the blender. Then I cut the top off and scooped out the flesh. It's a young coconut, so the flesh is really creamy. I added that to some frozen pineapple and the last of the fresh lime juice."

"So, what made it green?" Jenny asked.

"It's all about the greens, baby! A handful of kale, some romaine lettuce, and several handfuls of spinach."

"Wow," Jenny exclaimed, amazed that something with so much green in it could taste like a **Pina Colada**. "I've eaten more green stuff in the past twelve hours than I think I've eaten in a year. No wonder I'm feeling a little more – er, shall we say *regular?*"

The two women laughed.

"And is that why I also feel so awake?" asked Jenny, looking over at the clock which read 9 am. "I'll be honest with you, I'm usually still sleeping at this time on a Saturday morning."

Aunt Sue turned away from her task of note-taking to smile across at her niece. "Yes! It's amazing how quickly you'll feel the positive effects of getting some good green nutrition into your body, isn't it? I also wanted to make sure that last night's dinner wasn't just satisfying and filling, with probably something like ten times the nutritional value of what you'd normally eat, but that it was also relatively easy to digest. That way your body doesn't have so much work to do and can focus more on resting. Like a finely-tuned engine, your body performs better when it gets high-octane fuel that produces very little waste."

"I never thought of it that way before," said Jenny. "When I got up, my first thought was to make a cup of coffee and eat a bowl of cereal. Good thing I saw your note, because I figured I'd try your drink first. After that, I was so full and satisfied, and felt so completely awake that I didn't want or need anything else. To be honest with you, I don't much like the taste of coffee, but I drink it because it helps wake me up in the morning. I am getting hungry now, though, so maybe I should have just gone ahead and eaten the cereal. Is that what you do?"

Her aunt sprang up onto the kitchen counter, setting down the notepad and pen alongside where she sat. "I usually start my day with a big glass of water, often with a splash of lemon or lime and possibly some peppermint or lemon oil added, then I exercise and shower. I start my breakfast with a green smoothie similar to the one I made you earlier, or different, depending on what ingredients I have on hand, or freshly pressed green juice, and sometimes both," said Sue. "I sip on the smoothie or juice to fend off hunger while I make my breakfast. Some of my favorites for breakfast are **Chia Porridge, Cashew or Coconut Yogurt**, or sometimes my variation on Granola."

"Doesn't that take a lot of time?" Jenny asked.

"Well, it takes a bit longer than pouring cereal in a bowl, but not much! Over time, I've developed shortcuts that make it quick and easy. Especially if I do some advanced preparation. Would you like me to show you one of my favorite recipes, **Apple Ginger Medley?**"

Jenny nodded her assent as Sue jumped off the counter and began removing ingredients from the refrigerator and pantry. "This one's very quick and easy. I like it because it's not just delicious but really filling. Great if I have a busy day ahead or I'm going to be out shopping and know the only thing readily on offer is junk food. The nice thing about this recipe is that there are all sorts of variations I can do to keep it interesting, even if I eat it every day."

"Oh, I'm already an 'eat it every day' girl," laughed Jenny. "Only in my case it's Cornflakes with skim milk when I'm committed to dieting, and Cocoa Krispies with the full fat variety when I'm not."

"Well then Jenny, let's teach you how to make Apple Ginger Medley, and see what you think," said her aunt.

Five minutes later they were seated at the kitchen table enjoying this latest concoction from Sue, excitedly planning the day ahead. Jenny hoped she would remember how her aunt had made this latest breakfast.

Using Jenny's tiny food processor, she had chopped an apple with a one inch piece of fresh ginger and a handful of almonds that that had been left to soak overnight before they'd gone to bed. Placing this mixture in a bowl, Sue had poured in a tablespoon of lemon juice, added a pinch of cinnamon, a few drops of vanilla essence and a handful of shredded coconut. She then poured milk she'd made by blending a handful of raw macadamia nuts with water over the concoction, and then strained it into a pitcher to remove the pulp.

"I brought the macadamia nuts from home," Sue had explained. "I order them from a guy in Hawaii because they're so much tastier than the ones I can get at the market. They're freshly picked and he keeps them raw. Because they're harvested a week or two before he ships them out, they're still bursting with flavor when I get them. I store them in the freezer to keep them that way."

"Why did you soak the almonds overnight?" Jenny asked her aunt after they had moved out onto the patio to enjoy the warm morning air.

Aunt Sue explained that soaking and rinsing the nuts before eating them made them more digestible. She went on to explain about enzyme inhibitors and germination, topics that Jenny only partially understood.

"So what about last night when you made the fake tuna salad? You didn't soak the almonds then. Does that mean the tuna was harder to digest than our breakfast? Shouldn't you have soaked them then too?" Jenny asked.

"Ideally, yes, Jenny. But last time I checked life was not perfect, including the amount of time we have to rustle something up in a hurry. While I make a point to soak, rinse and drain my nuts before using them, it's not always possible. Years ago, when I was new to all of this, and I had all sorts of digestive issues, I had to be much more careful about it."

"How long have you been eating this way?" Jenny asked.

"Just over 10 years. Come to think of it, it must have been just after you and I last met. I'd been going through a rocky patch and had gained a lot of weight. I wasn't feeling especially well but couldn't put my finger on what was the matter. So I began doing some research and discovered the benefits of whole fresh foods, and how raw and living foods increase energy, help you lose weight, and even reverse disease. It sounded a bit odd and extreme to me, but I was intrigued. I read everything I could get my hands on, and the more I studied, the more I was drawn to it. I attended a three-week residential program that was just fabulous and life-changing for me. After that, there was no turning back. At the end of those three weeks, I felt better than I remember feeling in many years ... perhaps better than I'd ever felt in my entire life. My skin glowed, I was 20 pounds lighter and so full of energy. Part of the program involved some emotional cleansing to help support the physical changes. I'll be honest with you, it not only completely changed my life, but I'd go so far as to say it saved it too."

"Wow. Sounds amazing. But I'm not sure I'd just want to eat raw food. I like cooked stuff too much, especially when the weather gets cooler," said Jenny.

"Oh, it doesn't have to be all uncooked food, Jenny. It's more about balance. Raw and living foods certainly enhance how you look and feel and the more you eat, the healthier you tend to become. Some people start out trying one raw food meal a day; others make the change one hundred percent right away. Most people find that when about 75% to 80% of their food is whole, uncooked fresh plant-based food, their health blossoms. That way they've got some leeway for socializing or eating cooked foods when they want to. Each person needs to find the exact balance that works for them. For example, I'm really fond of steamed vegetables, especially broccoli, and I'm a sucker for the occasional baked sweet potato. Just not one that's oozing with butter."

Jenny sat quietly for a moment, soaking all of this in. Then she asked, "What's emotional cleansing?"

"Have you ever been a situation where you felt that a relationship was toxic to you, Jenny?" asked Sue. "I mean, when another person seems to be sucking the energy out of you, but you don't know how to change things?"

Patty's face popped immediately into Jenny's head and she remembered how despondent and pessimistic she tended to feel after their visits.

"Yes, uh, I do, I mean I am … yes … I've been in relationships like that, "Jenny stammered, hoping that her aunt wasn't going to ask for specifics.

"At the Center, I took part in a number of three-day juice fasts," Sue continued. "That meant drinking nothing but **Green Juice** for three days at a time - like kale, spinach, parsley, mint, which is my favorite - mixed with celery, cucumber and other highly nutritious ingredients. But aside from that, we attended classes that helped us get in touch with what lay at our core, such as our deepest goals and values. You'd be surprised at how many people go through life never considering these things, at least not until some crisis occurs, and sometimes not even then."

Jenny's aunt looked wistfully into the middle distance. After a few minutes of silence, she continued.

"After I'd worked through what was really important to me in life, I realized that some of the ways I was relating to people were actually toxic to me. I did a lot of writing - journaling - to express my forgiveness for the wrongs that had been done to me and apologies for my part in that dynamic. I resolved to be less judgmental and really open myself up to being fully present with others. By allowing myself to be vulnerable, I became more open to deeply loving and fulfilling relationships."

Jenny listened intently, realizing that there were so many facets to her aunt, and so many aspects of her own life that she had yet to explore. She suddenly felt a charge of energy, as if a glimmer of hope was coursing through her body. Then the thought came to her: what if she resolved to do everything that Aunt Sue did for their month together? Eating the same foods, exercising together, playing "follow the leader," in essence, with Aunt Sue as her inspiration? Might that help her break free from the dark cloud that seemed to be obscuring the light, making her life seem dull and gloomy in comparison?

"I haven't bored you to death, have I?" Aunt Sue asked, noticing that Jenny appeared deep in thought.

Jenny felt her aunt's hand on her own and was brought back to the present. "Not at all," said Jenny. "I was just thinking more about what you just shared and how I really want to break out of the funk of my life. Maybe if I almost become your clone, and do everything you do this month, I could experience the same sort of dramatic change?" Jenny felt her cheeks go red as she realized how desperate she sounded.

Her aunt leaned forward and looked deep into Jenny's eyes. "Sweetheart, you can make your life exactly how you choose. I'll be honored to share everything I know with you and guide you, if that's what you'd like. Certainly, I can provide you with the tools and the inspiration but it's up to you, ultimately, as to how you apply them. Just know that, for the next month at least, I'll be with you every step of the way."

Jenny felt an uneasy mixture of excitement and fear. She had so many questions; she didn't know where to begin. All she could think of to say was, "Aunt Sue, I've always been an A student. But I rarely learned anything of practical value in my life so I didn't always apply what I learned. This feels different, though. I truly believe that what you have to teach me has practical value."

Sue took Jenny's hand as she leapt out of her chair. "If it's practical value you're looking for, I know exactly where we can start." The older woman walked back to the kitchen, picked up the notebook and held it in the air. "I've been making a list of all the things you need, including a bigger, more powerful food processor."

Jenny opened her mouth to protest, but her aunt raised a finger. "No arguments. You've been such a good sport about letting me stay for a whole month, and I'm going to show my appreciation by getting you some kitchen tools. I've already ordered you a Vitamix blender, a water filter and a gadget you're going to love called a Spiralizer. They should arrive in the next week or so. The Spiralizer is great fun; it lets you make spaghetti out of zucchini.

"Hey, quit protesting," Sue continued, noticing the scowl on Jenny's face. "I get wholesale prices on everything through my company. I was on the Internet before I went running this morning; everything's set up. We can get the food processor locally."

Sue scanned her eyes over her notes. "What else? Yes, you need a good peeler, a food chopper, a citrus juicer, a serrated knife ... " Her voice trailed off as she looked around the kitchen. "Can't think of anything else right now, but if anything comes to me, we'll grab it later."

Jenny felt her eyes prick with tears. She offered up a croaky 'thanks' and hugged her aunt.

* * *

As she lay in bed that evening, Jenny mused on everything she had experienced. Her kitchen was about to become even more equipped with a variety of gadgets. Her Aunt Sue assured her they would be put to good use during the rest of their time together, and hopefully beyond.

The two women had gone shopping for a pair of new running shoes for Jenny, so they could start jogging together the next day. While looking at all the various brands and styles, Jenny learned that there was a great deal of science behind choosing the right footwear for your body and activity level.

Aunt Sue had advised her not to think about pushing herself by running on the trail, but to start out walking, and then a burst of running, followed by another short period of walking. "That way you can extend the running portion as you get stronger and your endurance builds," Sue assured her.

Jenny and her aunt had gone for a short walk to test the running shoes before dinner. While walking, Aunt Sue shared more information with Jenny — this time about a blood test that indicates whether or not a person is deficient in vitamin D. Jenny learned that sunscreen blocked her skin's ability to fully absorb the UV rays she needed to make Vitamin D in her skin. Sue had even suggested that a lack of Vitamin D might be contributing to the depression, fatigue and immune problems that Jenny had been suffering from intermittently since giving up the outdoor activities she used to take part in with Joy.

They had rounded off the day with what Sue had described as a "Mexican-Style Living Foods Meal" that had comprised of **Tacos** made with romaine lettuce tortillas, guacamole, salsa and "refried beans" made from cauliflower, sunflower seeds and sundried tomatoes.

Dessert was an **Apple Pie** that Aunt Sue took only minutes to conjure up, the crust being a wholesome blend of almonds, pecans and chia seeds to hold the filling brimming with chopped apples, cinnamon and a squeeze of lemon juice.

Jenny sighed contentedly. Change was coming; she could feel it. *Good change*. The kind of change she had been longing for, but just didn't know how to create for herself. Aunt Sue was a catalyst; the person she ideally needed to provoke her into making some fundamental changes in her life.

That was Jenny's last thought of the day. Within moments of deciding to make the changes she knew she was ready to make, she fell fast asleep.

CHAPTER 5

The Slippery Slope

Jenny nimbly navigated around the wrought-iron chairs and tables where fellow weekend visitors were eating meals, chastising unruly children, or serenely enjoying the view. She found an empty spot, set down her glass of Italian sparkling water, and began unlacing her walking shoes before slumping happily into her seat.

"I wouldn't think of taking those off until you get home, Jenny," Joy laughed, gesturing at her friend's feet before looking at her own. "How long were we out there? Three, maybe four hours? Oh, I'm so going to be soaking these babies when I get home."

"What about you, Aunt Sue?" Jenny asked. "How are you feeling?"

"Ready and willing for that triathlon I've signed up for. It's happening next weekend," the older woman said. "Thank you, ladies, for suggesting this. Just what I needed!"

Jenny nodded vigorously. "That was a fabulous hike. I'd forgotten how wonderful the right kind of exhaustion feels." The other women grunted in agreement.

"I can't believe we made it all the way to the top of Emerald Crest," Jenny continued, pointing to the peak in the distance. "If you told me a week ago that I'd be doing this, I'd never have believed you. What an accomplishment. Beats sitting around on the sofa eating chips and dip and watching movies!"

Jenny felt slightly guilty at disparaging her usual activities with Patty that she had turned down in order to make this trip with her aunt and best friend, but realized how much more beneficial the day had been - to her body, mind, and spirit.

"You were amazing, Jenny," said Joy. "To be honest, I was wondering if you'd be able to keep up with us, given that both Sue and I are exercise freaks! But we didn't have to slow down once. How did you do that?"

Jenny related to Joy how she had been staying true to her promise to eat mostly raw and unprocessed foods and to follow her aunt's guidance when it came to both nutrition and exercise.

"And doesn't she look absolutely radiant?" added Sue, squeezing Jenny's arm fondly. "I'm very proud of you, my dear."

The older woman turned to Joy. "And I'm especially delighted to have met you, Joy. Jenny has told me how much she's missed you recently." Joy smiled, turning toward Jenny.

"Now, Jenny - no need to blush, I don't think I'm speaking out of turn, here. You two are obviously close friends. It's important that you stay committed to that wonderful connection you each have."

Jenny leaned toward her friend and whispered in her ear, "I've missed you," before kissing her gently on the cheek.

She recalled how the two of them had made plans to visit Emerald Crest many times over the past year, but that she had always cancelled at the last minute, mostly because she just didn't have the energy to leave her apartment. This time, it was Jenny who had initiated the visit to their nearest state park.

"Wasn't this a great idea?" said Jenny. "And such a fantastic opportunity for two of the people I love most in the world to meet." She smiled broadly in the direction of Sue and Joy who were exchanging admiring glances.

"So what's been the result of eating all that green food your aunt's been feeding you?" laughed Joy.

"Well, I've already dropped eight pounds without any real effort on my part. And I'm finding I wake up before the alarm in the morning, although I still can't get that excited at the thought of going to work."

"Who can?" mumbled Joy, turning to Jenny's aunt who was sitting across the table from her. "Although Jenny tells me you love your work, Sue. Lucky you. I'd like to hear more about what you do. Sounds really interesting and value-creating."

"Maybe next time," said Jenny, shifting in her seat so she could pull out her cell phone from the back pocket of her shorts. After glancing at the screen, she added. "Time for us to go. I promised Patty I'd be ready to leave for the party by six, and I'm expecting traffic on the way home. Then I've got to shower and change before she picks me up. Sorry to cut our trip short, but I think we'd better leave now so I'm not late."

Joy looked at Jenny's aunt in unspoken agreement before saying, "Why don't you just leave the two of us here to enjoy the sunset? I hear it's spectacular on days like this. If that's okay with you, Sue?"

The older woman nodded in assent.

"That settles it then," continued Joy. "You go off and enjoy your party, Jenny, and I'll drive your aunt back when I've talked her into the ground."

"Sounds good to me, if that works for you Aunt Sue," said Jenny. "You're sure it's not too far out of your way, Joy?"

"Believe me, this is an opportunity I'm not going to miss!" said Joy. "You're not the only one who can learn something from your aunt. I need some major pointers on how to stop doing work I loathe. Maybe you can inspire me, Sue, to quit my job once and for all and find what it is I'm supposed to be doing with my life."

Sue beamed at the two younger women. "Oh, I think you give me way too much credit for changing your lives. Both you and Jenny have all the answers within you. But if I can help coach them out, then it'll be an honor."

"That settles it, then," said Jenny, scraping back the chair before bending down to tighten her laces. After checking that she had her cell phone and car keys, Jenny gave her aunt and best friend each a peck on the cheek and ambled back to the parking lot.

As she turned onto the main road home, Jenny heard her stomach rumble. She thought about how she had finished off the last of the energy bars her aunt had made, which they'd brought to snack on during their hike. With one hand on the wheel and the other fumbling sightlessly through her bag, Jenny realized she had nothing to eat.

"Oh well, I'll grab something quickly from the fridge when I get home," she thought.

The traffic was even worse than she'd imagined, and by the time Jenny got back to her apartment she barely had a chance to shower, get dressed and put on make-up - something she gotten out of the habit of doing altogether - before Patty arrived. Her friend didn't bother to ring the doorbell;

she walked straight in, while Jenny became acutely aware for the first time how that particular behavior bothered her.

As she closed the bedroom door behind her, Jenny noticed Patty staring at her from the living room.

"Is something the matter, Patty?" Jenny said.

"No," stuttered Patty. "It's just ... you look kinda ... uh ... different. Did you get a haircut or something?"

Jenny ran her hands down the side of the jeans she had been surprised to find now fit her comfortably, when just two weeks ago, they had been relegated to that part of her closet housing items for Goodwill. "Must be this new top my aunt bought me from that new boutique on High Street. Do you like it?"

Patty made an ambiguous sound before looking at her watch and saying, "Okay, no more time to chat. We'd better get our skates on. Don't want to ruin the surprise by walking in at the same time as the birthday girl."

Jenny looked into the kitchen, debating whether to stop long enough to grab another energy bar or smoothie.

"Come on!" Patty said, sounding irritated. "If you're needing food, there'll be plenty where we're headed. Can't wait. I've been looking forward to a big slice of chocolate birthday cake all day."

* * *

When Jenny returned from the bedroom where the party guests had been instructed to leave their jackets and bags, Patty was nowhere to be seen. Jenny found her minutes later in the dining room where a large table groaned under the weight of plates heaving with bowls of chips alongside creamy dips, cookies, platters with labels that reported "Breaded Fried Brie," "Mini Pork Sausages," and casserole dishes offering up "Cheesy Corn Bake," "Macaroni Cheese," and "Creamy Tuna Bake."

There were cheeses from different parts of the world, some oozing onto the plates from the heat in the room, others cut into bite-sized chunks. Jenny looked over and spotted Patty heaping a plate with a handful of crackers, then cutting a large wedge of what looked like sharp cheddar before heading toward the creamy casserole section of the table. Scanning the area for something that might be both nutritious and filling, Jenny spotted a tray of vegetable crudities - carrots, florets of broccoli and cauliflower, and short sticks of celery - decorously arranged around a bowl of thick, green-flecked, cream-colored dip.

This isn't going to be enough to get me through the evening, thought Jenny as she put a few carrots and sticks of celery on her plate and sampled the dip before deciding that she liked the taste of the spinach and cream cheese mix, and spooned a tablespoon of that on top of the vegetables. Jenny did another pass at the table, adding a sizeable portion of tuna bake before grabbing a bottle of water and looking around for a place to sit.

"Over here!" Jenny turned to see Patty beckoning her to join a group of women whom they both knew from their college days. After listening for ten minutes to the others discussing the food and complaining about their jobs and the men (or lack thereof) in their lives, Jenny used her empty plate as an excuse to get up and leave.

What downers, she thought as she negotiated her way back to the dining room, dancing around clumps of people who were either talking animatedly, or totally absorbed in eating and drinking.

"Wine or champagne?" someone holding a tray of drinks asked her, indicating that they would all be called upon to toast the birthday girl - another college girlfriend - very soon. Knowing that she wasn't the evening's designated driver, Jenny accepted a large glass of red wine. After several gulps, she became increasingly aware of how hungry she still was. Finishing the glass with a gulp, she headed back to the food table, and - rolling her eyes in recognition of her lack of will-power - she moved away from the vegetable platter, found a clean plate and began spooning small amounts of the various baked casseroles onto it, telling herself that if she kept to small quantities, it wouldn't disrupt her eating plan too much.

Then Patty was beside her. "Open wide," she ordered and Jenny's mouth willingly obeyed, her eyes closing in near ec-stasy at the delicious combination of crisp cracker and thickly- spread, creamy cheese topping.

Patty triumphantly propelled another cracker toward Jenny's mouth, but Jenny pursed her lips and shook her head. "That tasted great, but I've lost eight pounds and it feels really great to fit into these jeans. I'd better not."

Patty recoiled as if she had been slapped, and made a dis-paraging sound. "Oh, for goodness sake Jenny, don't start getting all *anorexic* on me. I mean, we've been looking for-ward to this party for months. What harm can one night do? I mean, if you can't enjoy yourself without feeling all guilty, you shouldn't have bothered coming."

Jenny's faced colored in annoyance and she suddenly be-came aware of how light-headed she felt.

"You might be able to squeeze into a smaller size of jeans, but you don't look all that great to me," continued Patty as she stuffed her own mouth with another cracker. After lick-ing her lips in appreciation, she said, "Well, it's up to you. Doesn't do to starve yourself, girlfriend. At least I know how to have a good time." Turning on her heels, Patty strode out of the room and into the melee of party guests.

Jenny didn't like the way she was feeling. She hated it when Patty got irritated with her, and this mixture of guilt and anger seemed to compound the unpleasant physical reactions Jenny was having to the alcohol in her bloodstream combined with hunger.

"Oh, to hell with it," she thought as she scanned the food table once more for dishes that were especially appealing, and began spooning larger amounts of gooey, calorie-laden foods onto her plate.

After finishing the food, Jenny helped herself to another glass of wine and felt the alcohol rush to her head as she joined in the raucous singing of "Happy Birthday." She could see Patty on the other side of the room, pointedly ignoring her. A hand glanced gently across her back, startling Jenny.

"Sorry, am I in your way?" she asked, then blushed as she looked into the deep blue eyes of a man she had noticed staring at her more than once, throughout the evening.

"Didn't mean to make you jump. Just wondered if you were up for a slice of birthday cake. I happen to find myself with two plates. Can't imagine how that happened," said the man, smiling flirtatiously. As Jenny accepted one of the plates, he held out his free hand. "I'm Max. I gather you're Jenny."

Jenny looked at him quizzically, "How'd you know my name?"

"I'm a mind reader," Max said, laughing at Jenny's startled look. "Just kidding. I overheard a couple of people talking about you - all good, I have to say - and thought it was such a nice name. I considered saying it was my mother's name, just to break the ice, but I wouldn't lie to you!"

Jenny and Max laughed in unison.

"So, how do you know the guest of honor?" Max asked.

"From college. She tutored me for a while when I was a freshman and she was in her senior year. You?"

"Neighbors. Actually childhood friends and neighbors," Max said, looking at Jenny in a way that felt deliciously unfamiliar.

She became aware of just how long it had been since a man had looked at her in any way that resembled interest. Jenny felt her stomach lurch, and wondered whether it was the effect of Max or the over-large amounts of cream and fat-laden food she'd just eaten. Her jeans were beginning to feel uncomfortably tight.

"Let me get you another glass of wine, Jenny," said Max, reaching for the empty glass in her hand and looking into her accepting eyes. "Is it the Merlot?"

The word "sure" was barely out of Jenny's mouth before Max took her glass and was off. Jenny suddenly felt vulnerable: lightheaded from the wine, but also nervous from Max's attention.

Jenny found him very attractive. She had always liked that look - tall, strong, dark hair and blue eyes ... similar to the physical traits of her father's side of the family.

What are you thinking? A voice inside her head chastised, sounding vaguely like Patty. *You're not ready for a man in your life. And anyway, he's just teasing you. A man that good looking can't possibly be serious. Don't let yourself get hurt. You know what men are like.*

Jenny suddenly noticed Patty bulldozing her way through the crowd.

"Wow, did you see that birthday cake?" she said, panting as she reached Jenny, acting as if nothing had happened between them. "Forty candles! Ugh. Remind me to leave the country on vacation when it's my turn. No surprise birthday parties for me, thank you very much."

Patty turned to face Jenny. "You okay?"

Jenny made a quick body assessment, as Aunt Sue had taught her to do. Her jeans were tightly stretched across her bloating stomach, and the combination of fat, sugar, and starch was wreaking havoc on her intestines. She realized she was not going to manage another glass of wine.

"Time to go home?" asked Patty, squeezing her friend's arm supportively.

"I think so," said Jenny, just as Max reached them, offering her the refilled glass.

"Sorry, gotta go," said Jenny apologetically.

"Yeah, I'm the driver and my car turns back into a pumpkin at midnight," added Patty as she grabbed Jenny's arm and began pulling her in the direction of the bedroom to collect their jackets.

Jenny wrestled her arm free and turned back to Max, holding out her hand.

"A pleasure to meet you," she said. "Thanks for the slice of cake. Better not to overdo it with the wine, though. Sorry for your wasted trip."

"No worries," Max shrugged. "Listen, can I get your number? I'd like to give you a call sometime in the week. Maybe we can grab a coffee together?"

"Oh, we don't give phone numbers to men we don't know," said Patty.

Max ignored her and looked directly at Jenny. "Well, look, here's my card with my number on it. Will you call me? I'd love to hear from you."

Jenny felt his hand press hers as she whispered "I will!"

Then he was gone.

Jenny stared at the card, aware of the unsettling mixture of disappointment and relief she was feeling. She was glad Patty had taken care of her nervousness about giving men her phone number, but she was also sorry that she'd not had the chance to get to know Max better.

Jenny was quiet during the drive home, tired of Patty's infernal chatter and grateful for the ability to tune her out as she watched other late-night travelers speed past in their vehicles.

"The nerve of that guy, asking for your number. You'd only just met him, right?" Jenny heard Patty say.

"Yeah," said Jenny, not wishing to start an argument. Left to her own devices, Jenny had a sneaky suspicion she would have gladly given him her number as he had requested. He was the first man in a long while who had showed any interest in her, but more importantly, she was definitely interested.

By the time Patty deposited Jenny at her apartment, she was too tired to think of anything other than the urgency of getting out of her jeans and into bed.

Sitting on the edge of her bed, Jenny sucked in her stomach as best she could before unzipping her pants, then looked down with dismay at the roll of flesh atop her panties. Feeling disappointed that she hadn't been able to resist the party food, Jenny was struck again by the bloating and heaviness she used to experience so regularly before Aunt Sue's arrival. One night of poor choices, and here she was nostalgic for the sense of lightness and comfort she'd known after exchanging her usual diet for Aunt Sue's delicious meals.

Her head pounding against her pillow, Jenny lay awake for a long time. She reached for the bottle of melatonin on her nightstand and realized that she hadn't taken any at all that week.

Her mind replayed the day as she took a gulp of water to wash the supplement down. The feelings of invigoration and pride as she completed the arduous climb to the top of Emerald Crest, with her aunt and Joy encouraging her on, were a sharp contrast to how she felt now.

"Darn it," she thought, as she drifted off to sleep.

CHAPTER 6

Training Wheels

"**A**re you okay?" Doris asked as Jenny walked past the office manager's desk on the way back to her cubicle. "I don't mean to be nosy, but it seems you've been spending a lot of time in the restroom this morning. And you look paler than normal. You're not sick, are you?"

Jenny didn't stop but called over her shoulder, "Thanks for the concern, Doris. Just a bit too much partying over the weekend." Back at her desk, Jenny rubbed her growling, distended stomach.

It's like a there's a rock in my intestines. I need some roto-rooter to unplug my pipes, she thought. She then moved her hands from her abdomen to her head, pressing each index finger against her temples in a vain attempt to ease the pain. She'd overslept this morning, and had missed Sue, who'd left her a green smoothie and a sweet note to say she'd be in meetings all day and would catch up with Jenny in the early evening after work.

Feeling bloated and puffy, Jenny had pulled on the kind of loose fitting skirt and top that the previous week she had been ready to discard forever at the Goodwill.

She had spent most of Sunday locked in her room, feigning menstrual cramps when Aunt Sue had knocked at her door at noon, concerned that Jenny hadn't gotten out of bed. Feeling sick and bloated, Jenny knew she could have claimed it was food poisoning from eating foods that had been picked at by many hands in an overheated room, but she knew the real reason for her discomfort. At the heart of it was her disappointment in herself, for making poor choices at the party. She was equally surprised at how quickly - and negatively - her body had responded. She definitely didn't feel ready to make this admission to her aunt.

"I'm not such good company the first day of my period. Since it's Sunday, I think I'll just stay in bed for a while longer," Jenny had explained, crossing her fingers on the other side of the locked door.

Jenny jumped as Professor Howell burst into her cubicle, bringing her thoughts abruptly back to the present. He waved a piece of paper in front of her face.

"I sent you an email first thing this morning asking you to prepare my monthly status report for the meeting at noon. How's that coming along? I need it urgently."

Jenny glanced surreptitiously at the clock on her computer screen. "I uh, was late getting in this morning ... been feeling a bit under the weather. Sorry. Haven't had chance to check my email yet."

"Oh, for goodness sake!" her boss exploded. "It's almost 11:30! You know how Monday mornings are around here. You didn't check your email? I rely on you to check it first thing in the morning for any urgent needs. This meeting was sprung on me this morning. I gave you three hours to do this, to free me up to prepare my presentation. It shouldn't have taken you more than an hour. Now you've got thirty minutes.

Get it to me by noon, Jenny, otherwise we're going to have that overdue talk."

Jenny closed her eyes and sighed, feeling like a very small child being scolded by a parent. "I'll get started right away, Professor Howell. Perhaps I can still complete it on time."

"Jenny, last week I was beginning to see glimpses of your old energy and competence. I started to think that perhaps you'd turned a corner. Seems that was a bit premature."

Jenny turned around to apologize once more, but her boss had already left in his now customary huff.

She quickly opened her email and saw the task Professor Howell had laid out. It wasn't as if she hadn't done this countless times before: compile statistics, lay them out in a spreadsheet, and include a few colorful graphical representations.

Jenny reached for her stress ball and gave it a tight squeeze. She took a deep breath and began reorganizing the numbers into a clear chart.

The clock on her computer showed 11:58 am as Jenny triumphantly hit the "send" button, report attached.

With the email now safely in cyberspace, Jenny felt inclined to re-read Professor Howell's original email, and realized with a sinking feeling that what he had asked for this morning was somewhat different than previous reports she'd prepared for him. Jenny slumped in her chair, feeling instantly sick to her stomach as she realized she'd omitted a critical section; the report was not going to fully reflect what he had asked for.

Jenny composed an apologetic email to Professor Howell, saying she was too sick to continue working that day. She hoped he'd accept that as the reason for her oversight, when the phone rang.

Her boss sounded colder than she had ever heard him. "The report you've sent me is incomplete, but I guess that's my problem. I've just sent to your printer a short list of additional data I need to carry this off. I was thinking of bypassing you altogether, Jenny, but you have the most direct access to this information. Please compile everything on that list ASAP, and come to the meeting room with it. I'll be seated at the back. I'm due to present in fifteen minutes." Then he hung up on her.

A concert of drums in her head, Jenny peeled the paper off the printer and struggled to focus. Aware of an increasing feeling of nausea, she rushed to collect the data Professor Howell had requested, then ran up three flights of stairs, arriving at the meeting room just as Professor Howell was stepping on to the stage. She waved the paper at him but he shook his head in response.

Now I'm really in trouble, Jenny thought as she slumped into the nearest chair. She didn't know whether to stay, in case Professor Howell changed his mind and required the material she had for him, or just leave and go home.

She sat there frozen, unaware of how much time had passed until the audience began clapping and Professor Howell began to gather up his papers. Jenny stood, and exited the stuffy room.

As she hurried to her desk, she felt the knot in her stomach tighten and expand, until it seemed as if it would choke her of breath. Hit with a fresh wave of nausea and lightheadedness, she headed toward the bathroom. She splashed her face with cool water and ducked inside the nearest stall. She sat down and began to sob.

Last week, she'd had a glimpse of what was possible for her, and now, Jenny bitterly resented how it had been snatched away. Avoiding both Professor Howell's office and Doris's desk, Jenny returned to her workspace and penned a quick note saying she needed to leave because she was sick. She shut off her computer, locked her desk and slipped away.

* * *

Back home, Jenny heard the front door of her apartment opening. She sat up with a start.

As Aunt Sue walked toward her, Jenny was struck by how energized and poised she looked, even after such a long work day. Sue sat down beside her niece, hugged her gently, and said, simply, "How was your day?" Jenny burst into tears.

"I think we need a cup of tea and a long chat," said Aunt Sue soothingly, patting Jenny's hand. Returning from the kitchen minutes later with two steaming mugs, Sue sat down on the sofa beside Jenny, listening as her niece spilled *everything* she'd been through, starting with the party and ending with her blow up with Professor Howell.

Sue held Jenny in silence until her sobs subsided, then placed her hands on top of Jenny's shoulders, looked into her niece's eyes and smiled. "Congratulations! You've discovered early on that you need to learn to crawl before you can expect to run. This is all very good! I know – that sounds crazy, right?" Sue laughed before continuing.

"Here's another crazy thought: let's get out of this apartment. There's nothing like a change of scenery, especially outdoors, to help put everything into perspective and reveal a clear way to move forward. It's a beautiful evening and I'm inclined to fix us a nice picnic dinner. Let's eat in the park, and we can talk more. Believe me, I understand what you've been going through! I have some stories I'd like to share with you. Let's get out of here!"

Barely half an hour later, the two of them were seated on a wooden bench overlooking the cycling path across from the park lake. The gleeful sounds of children enjoying the last hours of a balmy spring evening serenaded them as they opened the wicker basket and pulled out the boxes Sue had pulled together.

Sue pointed toward a group of people close by. "What do you see, Jenny?" Her niece looked over at a man in his late thirties or early forties, who was surrounded by a brood of children of various ages. A little girl happily rode her training bike in circles, keeping her eyes on the man the whole time. "She looks like she's afraid to take her eyes off Dad for very long, although he seems distracted by having to take the training wheels off that other bike and talking to his son," said Jenny. "The little boy is jumping up and down. I guess he's keen to just hop on and start riding."

Jenny and Sue watched silently as the small boy mounted the bike, his father holding on to the back of his seat while he started to peddle. "Let go, Dad," the boy was shouting as the bike wobbled from side to side.

"As soon as I feel you're balanced, I'll let you go," said his father. "It's all about balance, son. If you lean too far to either side, you'll topple over. Learn to keep your balance and you'll stay up just fine."

But the boy kept turning his head, urging his father to let him ride on his own. The man did as he was urged and released his grip, managing to run forward to save his son from hitting the pavement as the bike wobbled precariously.

"That was close!" said Jenny. "Good thing the dad was paying attention. The boy didn't have his balance."

Jenny and Sue were riveted by the scene unfolding in front of them. They watched as the father patiently worked with his son, letting go for a little longer each time, always managing to grab the bike again just before the boy fell off and hurt himself. Over time, the boy's skills improved. Then, the Dad let go, and the boy took off faster than the man could keep up. The bike went about ten feet before the son realized that his father was no longer alongside him, and he promptly toppled over.

The boy began to cry, "It's too hard. I'll never get it," he sobbed, as his father picked up both his son and the bike and headed back toward the other members of their family.

"I remember learning to ride a bicycle," said Jenny. "My dad told me that falling off was part of the process, and I just needed to keep getting back on. Each time, I'd stay on longer and longer. Then one day it just clicked and I never looked back."

Jenny smiled, feeling the light bulb illuminate over her head. "Is it the same with changing adult habits, Aunt Sue?" she asked. "If I keep getting back on track each time I fall off, will I eventually just stay on naturally?"

Aunt Sue reached across and squeezed Jenny's hand. "You've got it, my dear. Did you know that it takes at least twenty-one days to change a habit? That means you need to repeat a new habit over and over for three weeks before you start doing it unconsciously. After just a week of adopting new foods and habits, you're pretty much in the realm of "conscious incompetence," where you become aware of how much you suck at knowing what to do for your own good!"

Both women laughed.

Aunt Sue continued. "This is totally normal; I promise. As you develop more knowledge about what works and what doesn't, you can identify those moments when you're about to mess up, or have just done so. That's called 'conscious competence.' And eventually, with consistent focus and practice, you reach the state of "unconscious competence," when the new habit comes completely natural to you, just like riding a bike."

"I've never thought about it like that before," said Jenny wistfully. It made total sense. After a week of following Aunt Sue's lead, she was feeling so much better, but hadn't consciously applied that learning. When it came to embracing a completely new approach to food and well-being, Jenny was like the boy on the bike. Without a more experienced grip at the helm, Jenny had also lost her balance and had fallen back to her old ways.

"Tell me again what your father said to do when you fell off the bike, Jenny," Aunt Sue asked gently.

"He told me to get right back on and try again."

"Jenny, you still need training wheels, and that's okay! As you learn and grow, your balance will improve and you'll be able to move forward without them. But give yourself a break. What you're working on here involves some pretty major lifestyle changes. You've worked a long time to acquire these bad habits, and it's going to take some time to undo them."

Jenny nodded in agreement.

"And don't think any of us is exempt from this. I've got my own falling-off-the-bike story if you're inclined to hear it."

"Absolutely," said Jenny.

"Well, it was a doozy - quite the learning experience. It's like I tried to convey to you back in the apartment - often it's a blessing to fall off so early in the game, because it's then that you become more aware of what you need to do to set yourself up for success."

Sue lifted her feet onto the park bench and adjusted herself into a yoga position before continuing with her story.

"I already told you that once I spent three weeks at a fabulous spa retreat where I ate mostly fresh, living foods, exercised and meditated daily and ended up feeling really fabulous. When I went home, I did pretty well by myself for just over a month. My falling off moment happened at a close friend's wedding.

I was a member of the wedding party, and I hadn't voiced my dietary needs – nor did I think to take care of them myself. There I was, so busy with all the responsibilities I had, and because of that, I neglected my responsibilities to myself. First habit to go was preparing the green smoothie in the morning, even though I knew it offered me such a great start to the day.

Next, while in the bride's room taking photos and getting her ready for her grand entry, a waiter came in with a tray of hors d'oeuvres - the typical breaded and fried type, which, under normal circumstances, wouldn't have tempted me in the least. But I was starving and knew it would be hours before we sat down to dinner, when I had planned to eat a salad. So I nibbled on something ... can't remember exactly what ... fried shrimp maybe. I figured with all the good I'd done to my body over the last couple of months, one little appetizer couldn't hurt.

"But one appetizer turned into two, then three. There's something addictive about that type of food, you know? I later found out that it was probably the gluten in the coating that set off my food addictions. All the old cravings came back, big time."

"I so know what that's like," said Jenny, squeezing her aunt's upper arm gently.

"Then came the toast to the bride and groom, and I figured a little sip of champagne couldn't hurt. And it likely wouldn't have, but three glasses later, I was a mess! Suddenly, all my defenses were down, and I reverted right back to eating with reckless abandon, as I had done my entire life.

"Pardon the pun, but getting drunk like that was a sobering experience! Boy, did I feel sick the next day - not only physically, but also psychologically. The guilt and self-reproach were immobilizing. It took me several weeks to get back on track. Perhaps if there'd been someone I could have talked with, like you and I are doing now, then maybe things would have turned around for me sooner. But I had to work it out on my own."

"It's easy to think we're all alone in this," said Jenny. "I know so many women who think they can take a day off from their diet, especially at the beginning, because they fully intend to get back to the new regimen the next day.

"I've struggled with this most of my life. The day after, I typically come up with an excuse and make a promise to change that gets pushed back to the next day and then the next. It's usually a week or two before I become so disgusted at my weight gain that I vow to start again. Sometimes it's months before the urge to change kicks in. That's why I'm so grateful you're here, Aunt Sue. I did feel an immediate sense that I'd let myself down, and I know I need to get myself back on track, too. How did *you* do it?"

"The way I got myself back on track, Jenny, was to call the retreat center and make a phone appointment with one of their counselors. I'll never forget what she taught me."

"Which was? I'm dying to know," said Jenny.

"Remember our conversation shortly after I arrived? We talked about the importance of being connected to your big vision, your higher purpose. That's what I learned from that counselor. Most of us work on changing our diet and food habits from the perspective of *what we're doing*. What she taught me was the importance of changing *how we're being*, first. Once you change your mindset around who you are and how you want to be in the world, resulting action steps flow naturally. That really was a life-changing realization for me."

"I'm not sure I fully understand that," said Jenny. "Can you explain to me exactly what she taught you to do?"

The older woman smiled at her niece. "It takes a bit of time investment, Jenny, but it's well worth it. I found the talk with her so valuable that I signed up for a series of sessions in which she helped me get connected with my core values, and to set really juicy goals for myself. What was pivotal for me was not simply articulating the end result or outcome I wanted, like weighing a certain number of pounds less, but getting to the underlying *feeling state* that the result would offer me."

"I never thought about it that way before," said Jenny. "You mean, if I say I want to lose 25 pounds, that's not enough?"

"Precisely," said her aunt. "You have to know *why* that weight loss is important to you on an emotional level."

"Like, so I can feel good about fitting into all my old clothes?"

"Okay. But why is that so important to you, Jenny?"

Jenny sat quietly, thinking, before answering: "When I'm thinner and can wear clothes that fit me well and show off my fit and trim body, I feel attractive, I feel confident, I feel proud of who I am and ..." Jenny's voice trailed off.

"And what?" Aunt Sue encouraged. "When you feel attractive, confident and proud - what then?"

"I feel unstoppable. I'm clearer in my thinking, I perform better at my job, and I'm just plain happy."

"So! Let me put this another way. When you think about making a choice between, say, a piece of chocolate birthday cake and a plate of fruit, what would be a more compelling argument for choosing the fruit - losing the weight or feeling attractive, clear-headed, competent and happy?"

Jenny rolled her eyes and sighed. "That's just it," she said nodding. "When I try to motivate myself to do something based on losing weight, it always feels like a deprivation. When I think about doing something because it makes me happy, competent and clear-headed, I feel inspired."

"Exactly," said her aunt, beaming. "You got it! And here's another thing I learned from my mentor: the actual language you use is all-important, because your subconscious "hears" words differently than you might have meant them. For example, what comes to mind when you think about losing something that belongs to you?"

Jenny shrugged. "I guess my first thought is to look for it, to find it. But when I lose weight I don't want to get it back."

"Right!" said Aunt Sue replied. "But the message your subconscious receives is that you've lost something that now needs to be found, which in turn triggers the thoughts, feelings and actions that direct you to finding that lost weight."

Sue uncapped her flask of water and took a long drink before continuing. "How many weight loss programs have you tried, Jenny? Two, three, more?"

Jenny shook her head. "Dozens!"

"Right! You and half the adult female population. My mentor taught me to think of dieting as letting the weight go. Getting rid of the extra pounds. Once I changed my mindset, my actions began to flow effortlessly."

"Wow. This is so helpful," Jenny said, hugging her aunt.

"There are a number of exercises I learned that I'd be happy to share with you, Jenny, if you're ready to get off the rollercoaster."

"I'm more than ready. But I do have another question, Aunt Sue, more of a practical one. How do you handle going to parties or events when there really are no healthy options to choose from?"

"You need my **Healthy-Eating-on-the-Run Survivors Guide!**" Aunt Sue replied. I actually wrote an article about this very topic, and I created checklists for an online magazine a while back. Remind me to send you the link when we get home. But here's tip number one, which may at first seem counterintuitive: never go to a party - or restaurant, for that matter - when you're feeling hungry.

"Part of the reason your guard was down the other night was because you were starving. Remember, we'd hiked all day and those energy bars we'd eaten on the way down from the peak couldn't sustain you for that long period of time. You were in a rush to leave and hadn't had time to eat, so you were already vulnerable when you arrived."

"That makes sense! So what would you have done, in the same situation, Aunt Sue?"

"I would have been late to the party, taking the time to make something nutritious and filling, like a smoothie. I probably would have stashed a green energy bar in my purse, so that if there really was nothing there to eat, I could sneak into the bathroom and nibble on it. Usually when I go to a party, I plan in advance and make a dish to contribute to the spread. That way, I know that there will be at least one nourishing thing I can eat. Besides, most hosts really appreciate it when you bring something."

"I never thought of that," said Jenny.

"I used to always carry food with me," Sue continued. "I've been doing this for so long now, it's second nature - unconscious competence again - and if I DO find myself in a position where I don't have something nutritious with me, I just ignore the hunger until I get home. Things don't tempt me the way they used to anymore. But in the early years, I was *always* prepared. After going through the six-week food binge that followed the wedding I told you about, I wasn't willing to risk experiencing that ever again."

"It seems like a lot of work to have to always prepare food when you go out," said Jenny.

"Yes, I can see how you might think that. But let me ask you this: How long did it take me to pull this delicious picnic together? Ten minutes? Twelve tops? I think it's fun, looking in the fridge for things to throw together for a fast meal. It's a never-ending adventure, Jenny, and having fun while you do it is more than just a big part of the process. It's actually critical to your success. If your new habits are not fun, you'll soon revert back to the old ones that you feel are."

"I wish I could just take some time off and really immerse myself in this, like you did when you went to that retreat. I'm sure I'd have more fun being in the kitchen once I'd learned a few tricks. I'm so sick of my job right now, of my boss, and the stress of messing up all the time. I haven't had a vacation in so long and ..."

Sue interrupted her, "Darling, I have an idea. Take next week off. I've got the race on Sunday, and I always reward myself with a day of pampering afterward. I was thinking of visiting the Lakeside Day Spa on Monday, but even better, I believe they've got some overnight specials they're offering at the moment, and it would be so fun to go together!"

Sue reached into her pocket and pulled out her cell phone. She punched in a number and after a brief conversation, turned to Jenny and said: "They can accept us for a three-night package starting Monday. Massages, facials, swimming, great food, hiking - the works! Seems the place is fairly quiet right now, so if we love it, we can even extend our stay for the whole week! All you have to do is let that bad-tempered boss of yours know that he's going to have to live without you for a bit. Deal?"

Jenny was speechless.

"Oh, and it's my treat, in case you are worried about the cost. Another way I can thank you for putting up with me for so long."

"It's hardly a punishment, Auntie," said Jenny, rapidly considering whether she should throw caution to the wind and claim vacation, or just call in sick.

Her aunt nudged her elbow gently into Jenny's ribs. "Well, what do you say?"

"My boss won't like it, but I love the idea!" exclaimed Jenny. "I have vacation time left over from last year that I didn't take, and I'll lose those days if I don't claim them soon. Plus, I can't think of anyone I'd most like to spend quality time with than you."

Jenny hugged her aunt and said, "Yes, let's do it!"

"Ok, then it's settled. I'll call them back and book it, and you deal with that dreadful boss of yours."

Jenny hugged her aunt, her eyes filling with tears as she said softly, "You are the answer to my prayers. Thank you so much for being here and being you, Aunt Sue. One thing's for sure: I won't let either of us down again. I promise."

CHAPTER **7**

Race Day

Jenny held the phone away from her ear as her friend shouted. "Yes, I know, Patty, we haven't found time to get together on Saturday in a while, but I just can't do it tomorrow either," said Jenny, as soon as she was able to get a word in edgewise. "I need to work part of this weekend. I'm taking some time off next week and promised Professor Howell I'd finish a couple of small projects before I go. There was no way he was going to agree to me taking vacation time otherwise."

"How about Sunday, then?" snapped Patty. Feeling guilty, Jenny couldn't think of any reason to say no to her, although she was not looking forward to a day of just sitting on Patty's sofa, watching TV, eating chips and complaining about work.

"Aunt Sue will be busy in the morning with her race. Why don't we get together then?" Jenny listened for the assent from her friend and said, "Right. See you Sunday around ten, then."

Jenny set down the receiver and walked back to the dinner table, hoping the homemade sorbet she had been about to enjoy when Patty called hadn't melted too much.

"Did I hear you make plans for Sunday, dear?" Aunt Sue inquired, peering up at Jenny over the top of the magazine she was flipping through.

"Yes, why?" Jenny asked, detecting a note of disappointment in Sue's voice.

"That's the day of my race, Jenny. I was looking forward to you cheering me on. You've got an important role to play, handing me snacks and water along the route."

"You don't really need me to do that, do you? I mean, there are water stops and volunteers who will help with that, right?"

"Jenny, that's not the point. It is so much nicer to have a familiar face at these events. It's more motivating and inspiring. Usually, in my hometown, I have a friend cheer me on. I know we hadn't made any definite plans. I guess I was just expecting you to be there."

Jenny blushed and gripped her silverware more tightly.

"Sorry, Aunt Sue. It's just that I haven't spent the day with Patty in a long time, and she was pressuring me, so I thought ..."

"Then invite her along," Sue interjected. "After all, I'm sure you'd both like a change. The weather is supposed to be spectacular! You could both soak up the sun before it gets too hot."

"I'll do that now," said Jenny as she got up from the table to retrieve her phone.

"You can tell Patty from me that it's a really fun, empowering event, even for spectators," Sue called to her from across the room. "You'll get to see folks with disabilities as well as cancer survivors who are raising money for charity. Would you believe many of the triathletes are even older than me? The last race I took part in, the oldest participant was a 94-year-old great-great grandmother. Can you believe that?"

Jenny smiled, realizing with excitement how fun the race might be.

A few minutes later, she was back at the dining room table.

"Patty said no."

"That was quick call," said Sue, placing the magazine back on the table and looking up. "You look upset, dear. Sounded to me like you had some kind of argument."

Jenny sighed. "Patty says I've changed and have no time for her anymore," Jenny grimaced. "But most of her anger is aimed at you, Aunt Sue."

Sue threw her head back and laughed heartily. "That's quite alright, my dear! When you begin improving yourself, sometimes those around you aren't ready for change. Sometimes, they might even resent you for moving forward without them."

Sue got up and began to remove the dinner dishes from the table and place them in the dishwasher.

"So," she asked casually, turning on a faucet to rinse off the plates. "It's just you and me at the race tomorrow. Or do you feel you need to be with Patty?"

"After that conversation," said Jenny. "Absolutely not. Patty is in a rut and seems intent on keeping me there with her. I don't want to end our friendship, but I can't let it keep going the way it has been. What I want out of life has changed - pretty much since you arrived, Aunt Sue. And that's a good thing. The trouble is, I don't know how to talk to Patty about it. She's just so confrontational."

"Support systems are the key to success," said Sue, as she placed the handful of silverware that she had just rinsed under the running water into the dishwasher. "The important thing is to surround yourself with people who lift you up. Like Joy, for instance. She's a keeper, Jenny. I've seen how much she really cares about you. I wonder if you can say the same about Patty, who seems threatened by the new you. She's afraid you'll leave her behind but seems unable to do anything about her fears. But that's her issue, Jenny, not yours. I doubt there's anything you can do about your friend until she reaches out and asks for help, just as you did with me."

Jenny pondered Aunt Sue's words, realizing it was all about commitment. The more Jenny had fully committed to a lifestyle that lifted her spirits, the more she needed to surround herself with people who were willing to be supportive companions on her new journey.

$$* * *$$

The hot sun felt so good on Jenny's bare arms, as she looked out over the sea of bicycles being ridden by people of every shape, size and age. The air was thick with the sounds of cheering supporters, and the aroma of various foods ranging from barbecued meats to cotton candy. Jenny looked at the route plan Aunt Sue had given her earlier, then at her watch. Sue would be passing by in roughly ten minutes.

Gazing at the athletes whizzing by, Jenny was startled by a hand squeezing her shoulder and a voice whispering "Hey, there," in her ear.

Jenny turned to stare into a familiar handsome face, and bright blue eyes.

"Max!," she breathed, "You scared me half to death!"

"Serves you right. You didn't call me like you said you would," Max said with a chuckle. His face changed to one of mock sadness. "And you didn't intend to, did you? I was hoping that you would but I didn't think so. Your friend was intent on getting you away from me as fast as she could. I figured she'd given you a lecture about calling strange men you meet at parties."

Jenny blushed. "I was going to, honest. But I took ill right after the party and then, I guess ... I guess I just forgot. I'm sorry."

"Sounds like I didn't make much of an impression on you," Max said in self-mocking tone. "But I'm sorry to hear you were ill. Too much alcohol?"

"And chocolate cake and cheese and creamy dips ... everything. I'd been on a mostly raw food diet for about a week before the party and that was extreme overindulgence ... for which I paid the price."

"Raw food, huh? That sounds cool," said Max. "I've been thinking about looking seriously at my diet for a while. Maybe you could share what you know with me?"

"Sure, glad to, although it's my Aunt Sue who's been staying with me who's the real expert. Unfortunately, she's only here for another couple of weeks. But I've learned enough to be helpful, I think!" Jenny said, becoming aware of how different she felt and acted in this man's presence. "My aunt should be coming around the corner any time now. What about you? What are you doing here?"

Max uncoupled a water container from his belt and took a long drink before responding. "Oh, I'm a volunteer. Do it every year. My thing is helping the disabled athletes in the transition area. I call it the Formula One Pit Stop - you know, helping them re-fuel with fresh water, some fruit to keep their energy level up, make sure their equipment is working properly, that kind of thing. They inspire me with their dedication and focus. It's an honor to be part of something like this."

"You don't race, then?"

Max rubbed his left knee. "Old war wound. Cartilage problems from playing too much football in my youth. Nowadays I find it healthier to contribute from the sidelines. How about you? Ever thought of taking part yourself?"

"Not up to this point," said Jenny. "My inspiration is my aunt, so I might sign up for next year. But I seriously need to get my body in shape before I dare get into running gear."

Max cocked his head to one side and looked at her approvingly. "Seems to me you'd look great in running gear."

Jenny felt her cheeks turn from sun-dappled pink to deep red.

"Thanks, "Jenny spluttered, unsuccessfully willing the color in her face to go away.

"Tell me more about the disabled racers, Max," she said, hoping that a change of subject would make her feel less uncomfortable, although it was - to her surprise - a pleasant discomfort. "How do they manage such physically demanding activities?"

"Where there's a will, there's a way, Jenny. Some use wheel chairs, others have specially- designed cycles. They're determined and positive, and ..." Max glanced at his watch. "... And I see one of them right now. Jenny, I hate to run off like this, but I need to go. Can I call you later - once the race is over? That is, if you don't already have plans? I'd love to take you and your aunt for a bite to eat. I heard that a new organic restaurant just opened up over on the east side, and they serve raw foods and other healthy fare. You think she would be up for that?"

Jenny looked directly into Max's warm blue eyes. She could tell from the way they twinkled that this was a guy who would be really fun to get to know.

"I'm sorry, Max," Jenny began.

"Uh-oh here it comes," Max interjected. "Another let down. Just be gentle with me."

Jenny laughed. She couldn't remember laughing so much with a man in quite some time. She gently nudged his ribs with her elbow. "What I was *going* to say before you so rudely interrupted me is that I'm not sure what time my aunt will finish, or what she has in mind after the event is over. But, yes, I'd love it if you'd call me. Let's check in with each other in a bit, ok?"

Max grinned, rummaged in his pants pocket and pulled out an old receipt and a pencil. "Write down your number for me," he said, and Jenny did.

"Gotta run ... don't want to be late. Great bumping into you, Jenny. I'll call you around noon."

Jenny could feel a long-forgotten, warm feeling suffuse her body. She was still smiling when she heard her aunt's voice calling out from among the throng of cyclists heading her way.

Jenny waved and cheered as her aunt skidded to a halt in front of her. Jenny took out a homemade energy bar from the bag she was carrying, and as her aunt began devouring it, Jenny poured her a cupful of green juice from a vacuum flask. Sue looked at her in appreciation. "Boy, this is fun. See you at the next stop," Sue said before handing the cup back to Jenny, positioning her right foot on the pedal and pushing off.

Jenny watched her aunt disappear amid the cyclists, then pulled out her map to be sure she knew where to be standing when her aunt arrived at the next station. She looked at her watch. 10:20. Less than two hours to go before Max was due to call her. Jenny grinned all the way to the next pit stop.

* * *

"How do you feel?" Jenny asked her aunt at the finish line.

"Absolutely marvelous, darling," said Sue, her hair plastered to her head and her skin glistening with sweat. "And I'm particularly delighted that I shaved off so much time from my last race! Always good to see improvement. What time is it, dear?"

"Eleven-thirty. Listen, Aunt Sue, I'm going to be getting a call from a new friend of mine - Max - in about half an hour. He's a volunteer here and was wondering if he could take us both out to eat. I didn't make a definite commitment because I thought you might be too tired and not feel up to it ..."

"Oh, I'm sure he doesn't want me coming along, but it was polite of him to invite me anyway."

"Well, I can't say what he wants, but I want you to be there!"

"What? You don't want to be with this guy alone?" said Sue, hands on her hips and breathing deeply.

"Actually, I like him ... well, what I've seen so far, I like. It's just that it's been such a long time since any guy asked me out ..."

"And you want me to be your chaperone?" Sue laughed. "You are funny, Jenny. Tell me, what does this young man have in mind?"

"I'll know more when he calls. But he said something about a new raw food restaurant he'd like to try."

"Sounds like my kind of arrangement. Come on, my dear. Let's get out of this zoo so we can get cleaned up and ready for "our" date! What did you say your friend's name is?"

"Max." As she said his name, Jenny felt a warm glow of contentment. It would be good to see him again.

* * *

"So, Max, what do you do?"

The trio had just been seated in a booth by a heavily tat-tooed waitress who, rather than handing them menus, pointed up at a huge chalkboard boasting all sorts of deli-cious-sounding fare.

"I'm your typical techie, Sue," answered Max. "Work for a software company here in town. Very boring stuff, but I'm good at it and it pays really well. I've given myself another three or four years - then I'm out of there. I want to develop online training to help people with disabilities take ad-vantage of social media. So many of the folks I've met since volunteering at races have great ideas for home-based small businesses, but just don't know how to market and promote themselves online. That's something I've become pretty good at, so I was thinking of starting my own business. I think there's a big future in this line of work. More to the point, it's where my heart is."

Max looked over at Jenny and smiled. She felt something lurch in her chest, as if her heart had just turned a joyful cart-wheel.

"Sounds like you've got it all figured out," said Sue, taking a sip of water.

"Can any of us ever say that?" said Max. "I have a vision for my life and I'm developing the skills I need to make it a reality. But who knows what could come up? I like to leave enough room for uncertainty, because that's when the real gifts come to you."

The waitress interrupted them to take their order. When she had left, Max turned back to Jenny and said, "How about you? D'you plan to stay at the university long-term?"

"I guess so," said Jenny, aware of Sue looking quizzically at her and adding, "Well, not if I won the lottery or anything like that. It's secure employment, so at least I know my rent will get paid every month." Jenny colored up as the others stared at her, seemingly astounded by this revelation. "I mean, in these times, that's not so unreasonable, is it?" she blurted.

As if sensing that Jenny was feeling backed into a corner, Max asked Sue about her work.

Jenny's aunt entertained them during the first part of the meal with her "stories from the trenches," as she described them. The mood had lightened considerably by the time the trio was dipping spoons into the two desserts that had been placed in the middle of the table so that each of them could have a taste of their favorite picks - a raspberry-orange sorbet, and a no-bake, wheat-free, low-glycemic vanilla and organic chocolate cheesecake.

Sue nudged Max conspiratorially. "You know, Max," she said, winking at him, "I think Jenny is due for a change from that dull university job. Don't you agree that she has so much more to offer than being an administrative assistant for an academic?"

"I would certainly say so," Max agreed, playing along by lowering his tone as if there were a secret between him and the older woman. "But what else do you think she might want to do?"

"Let's ask her," said Sue brightly. "Jenny - imagine you never had to worry about money ever again. Imagine getting up each morning and doing exactly what you wanted: the only proviso being that it must add value to the world. No sitting around lounging on a Jamaican beach all day, sipping rum and having your feet manicured."

The three of them laughed in unison.

"Yes, Jenny," said Max. "Let's pretend! It's so much easier to fire the imagination up when you're not weighed down by worries about paying your rent, or how you're going to feed the cat, or whatever."

He instructed Jenny to close her eyes and picture herself in, say, six months or a year's time. He asked her what she was doing to make a contribution. He asked her what was in her heart, as opposed to her left brain.

Jenny put down her spoon, dabbed the sides of her mouth with her napkin and sat back in her chair, extending her feet, aware that one of them was nestled close to Max's under the table. He didn't move his away and neither did she. Jenny closed her eyes, and took a deep breath, as Sue has taught her to do when she was about to go quietly within.

The restaurant, which had been thinning out with diners, seemed to go quiet. Within moments, Jenny felt tears prick her eyes. As she blinked, a single tear rolled down her right cheek. She captured its saltiness with the tip of her tongue, smiled and opened her eyes.

The first thing Jenny saw when her eyes re-focused was her aunt's worried face.

"Oh, my dear Jenny," said Sue. "We didn't mean to upset you."

Jenny shook her head vigorously and extended her hand to squeeze her aunt's arm. "I'm not upset, auntie. It was wonderful - so clear and moving. I've never had an intuition like that in my entire life."

After a moment's silence Sue said, "I'm dying to know. Can you tell us what you saw - or is it too private?"

Jenny looked across the table at Max who appeared as equally interested as Sue. He raised an eyebrow and squeezed his lips together in a way that, again, made Jenny's heart lurch in her chest. She instinctively reached for his hand.

Jenny began, "I was sitting outside in this beautiful natural place, up in the mountains I think. I was surrounded by all these excited young people and they were eating and giving me compliments. I think I must have prepared a picnic for us all." Jenny looked across at Max and Sue who nodded for her to continue.

"But I got the sense that this was more than a social occasion. Like, food – preparing it, serving it - was a big part of my life. But not in a restaurant or anything like that. It was hard to make sense of it really. I just know that I felt such intense pleasure."

Jenny paused and took a deep breath. "Food, fun, and friends. I think that's what my future life is going to be all about. Can't tell you any more details than that, except that I think maybe I'm supposed to look into getting some sort of culinary school qualification. Changing my relationship with food, thanks to Aunt Sue here, has done wonders for my life. I'm thinking I want to do something similar for others. I don't know – maybe I'll end up being some kind of food coach or something? But I'd really like to combine that with nonprofit work. I have no idea how that's going to come together," Jenny laughed.

"Wow, Jenny, you sound really energized! There's a whole world of possibilities there. Good for you!" said Max when Jenny picked up her spoon to finish off the last bite of cheesecake. Sue nodded in agreement.

Jenny couldn't remember three hours ever having passed so quickly. The conversation never waned, and she loved those moments when Max would reach across and touch her hand or grab her arm gently to emphasize the point he was making. From time to time, she would steal a glance at her aunt, too, who either winked approvingly, or surreptitiously nodded her head.

* * *

"Well, what did you think of Max?" Jenny felt the question was redundant even as she spoke it, but she wanted to keep the conversation focused on him, as the two women journeyed home.

"I like him! I hope you're planning to see him again when we get back from the spa. Once I'm out of your hair, you'll have plenty of time for dating," said Sue. "I saw you two huddling together at the end. It was so cute! It's obvious he likes you. But what about you? How are you feeling?"

Jenny blushed. "He seems really nice. And he makes me laugh, which is always a delight."

"You know, one of the things that impressed me most was when he talked about his work. Not so much what he's doing now, but what he intends to do in the future," said Sue. "It always impresses me when someone realizes that what they're doing meets their financial needs, but not their intellectual or spiritual needs. I think he's a very sensible young man to pre-empt a mid-life crisis like this."

"What do you mean?"

"Well, you're too young to appreciate this at the moment, but for so many people, there comes a time when they realize that the ladder of success they've been so focused on climbing is actually up against the wrong wall. That they invested so much of themselves in a profession that they just stumbled into, or that someone - like a parent or career counselor - suggested to them was *suitable*, when they should have run screaming for the hills and done what their heart told them to do, instead.

"Life is way too short, Jenny, to be working for an organization or a boss who fails to inspire you to greatness. If you're just going through the motions, what does that say about your commitment to your life?"

The two of them were quiet for some miles before Sue spoke again.

"So, my dear. Off to our next adventure! Tomorrow we go to the spa and allow our bodies, minds and spirits to be pampered. Maybe that would be a good time for you to think more about that picture you saw of a new future: one that's different from your past *and* your present. Isn't that exciting?"

Jenny just smiled. She wasn't ready to share what she was thinking: that a future with a deep, sensitive, lovely man like Max would be blissfully different, indeed.

CHAPTER 8

A Blessing in Disguise

"It's amazing what a week off has done to my attitude, Aunt Sue! I feel so well-rested and happy! Even the prospect of being back at the office in an hour from now isn't bothering me." Jenny savored the **Lime Mint Smoothie** her aunt had just handed her before setting the glass down on the kitchen table.

"Not to say I told you so," Sue replied, "but taking care of yourself for a week really does give you a whole new perspective on life, doesn't it?"

Jenny nodded in assent as she set a bowl down in front of her Aunt. "Here, try this. I followed your recipe exactly, except for a little extra cinnamon and a bit of vanilla."

"It's delicious," the older woman responded, as she savored a spoonful of the **Coconut Chia Pudding** Jenny had prepared earlier. "I'm impressed by how good you've become at rustling up these wonderful meals. You're quite the little food preparer now."

"Hardly 'little' yet, Auntie, but I'm getting there. I've dropped another four pounds since we got back from the spa, and my pants are feeling looser." Jenny held out the waistline of her jeans to show her aunt the extra space between her belly and her pants. "And I love how much lighter I feel, not just in my body. I'm determined to make this a way of life from here on. There's no turning back for me now."

"I'm so proud of you! Now, I need to run, my dear," said Sue as she gathered up her car keys and the two folders lying on the sideboard next to the front door. "Should be back for dinner around six or so. Anything you need me to pick up on the way home?"

Jenny shook her head and Sue hugged her niece tightly. "Have fun at work today, Jenny. Remember what we talked about last week. Your attitude makes all the difference in the world. And try out that little energy projection technique we learned at the spa. It just might help out with that boss of yours."

"He's probably beyond help, but I'll certainly try," Jenny joked as she waved her aunt out the door.

"Remember Jenny, it's not about 'try,' it's about 'do'!"

* * *

"How was your week off?" Doris called out as Jenny sauntered past the office manager's door.

"Fabulous!" said Jenny, leaning against the door frame. "I haven't felt this good in a long time."

Doris looked at her awkwardly as if, for the first time, she hoped Jenny wouldn't stand there chatting for long.

"What's been going on here while I've been away? Same old, same old?" Jenny asked.

"Not really," said Doris, looking at her computer screen and beginning to type. "Sorry, but I need to attend to this email. Catch up with you later. Glad you had a good time away."

Jenny shrugged. It was typically she who cut short their conversations, but she was looking forward to getting to her workstation to see what projects were waiting for her. She walked down the corridor, smiling at her co-workers, who she noticed looked even more stressed-out and worn down than usual.

"Jenny, we need to talk." Professor Howell appeared at her workstation just as Jenny was turning on her computer.

"Sure thing, Professor," Jenny said, beaming up at her boss. He gestured for her to follow him into his office. Jenny threw her purse under the table and grabbed a lined pad and pen from the top drawer of her desk.

"Well," Jenny beamed as she sat in the swivel chair opposite her boss in his book-lined office. "I'm sure there's a long list of projects just waiting for me to start on. Thanks again for letting me take last week off with such short notice. I feel really rested now, and am ready to get back on top of things."

"Well, Jenny. That's not exactly what I had in mind," said Professor Howell, ominously.

* * *

"Another successful day out of the way," Aunt Sue exclaimed as she burst through the front door of Jenny's apartment.

She stopped midway to the guest bedroom and inhaled deeply. Diverting to the living area, she found Jenny and Joy sitting knee-to-knee on the couch. "Smells like you girls are having a party. Hope that's organic red wine," Sue joked, glancing at the half-filled bottle and two glasses atop the coffee table.

"Okay. Who died?" Sue asked solemnly, when she saw the dark circles and puffiness under Jenny's red-rimmed eyes.

"No one", Jenny answered, tearing up. "I got fired."

Aunt Sue paused for a moment, then threw her arms into the air in an expression of triumph. "Congratulations!"

Jenny and Joy looked at the older woman as if she'd lost her mind.

"Didn't you hear what she said? Jenny has lost her job," Joy said, adding sarcastically, "I don't think congratulations are in order."

"I disagree, Joy. Congratulations are exactly what's called for," Aunt Sue repeated. "You're lucky indeed when your boss is so supportive of your new life that he fires you."

"Oh, come on Sue," Joy responded. "Is now really the time for your relentless positivity? I'm all for seeing the silver lining, but now is not the time. Can't you see that Jenny is upset? She's been crying for hours. She lost her job. It's serious, and we need to help her to figure out what's next."

Sue sat down on the couch beside Jenny. She put her arm around her niece and hugged her tight. "I know it feels like your world is caving in right now, honey. And I get how the uncertainty you're feeling about your future is driving you to seek old comfortable behaviors," she said pointing to the half empty bottle of wine. "But all you need is right here." The older woman touched Jenny's head and heart simultaneously. "You were standing at the edge of the cliff, too afraid to jump into the water below. Your boss just gave you a push in the direction you were destined to head! Maybe you weren't quite ready, but the water feels great once you're in it for a while."

Jenny blew her nose loudly into the tissue that Joy handed her, as Sue continued.

"Jenny, you know you weren't happy working at the university. How much longer would you have stayed on, trying to make it work when your heart wasn't in it? All the while having the stress and pain of your unfulfilled desires eating away at you, throwing a monkey wrench into your healing progress, and detrimentally impacting even the best diet and exercise plan."

"I get all that, Aunt Sue," Jenny said in a whisper, her voice croaky from all the talking and crying. "But I can't pay the rent with passion. The job may not be ideal for me, but it's food on the table. And this couldn't have come at a worse time. You're leaving in a few days and I'm scared that I'll just fall apart without your support."

"How much do you have in savings, Jenny?" interrupted Joy. "How many months can you live on your savings if you need to?"

"I don't know for sure," Jenny replied, her sharp mind for figures automatically beginning various mental calculations.

Their conversation was interrupted by the ringing of her cell phone. She glanced at it to see who was calling, and felt a tightening in her throat along with a flutter of excitement in her chest. Instinctively, she pressed the 'talk' button and began to speak, hoping that her voice wouldn't reveal her upset.

"Hi Max," she choked into the phone.

"Jenny, it's great to hear your voice," said the Max on the other end. "Hey, look, I'm headed in your direction and would love to take you bowling. There's a little tournament ... the kids group I was telling you about - you know, the kids with disabilities. It would be a great way for you to find out firsthand about the group I volunteer with. The kids are a delight to be around ... so determined and positive, in spite of their handicaps. And many of them usually kick the pants off me at bowling! Wanna join us?"

"Max, uh, normally I'd love to. But I've had some bad news today."

"Oh, gosh, I'm sorry," said Max. "I hope it wasn't, like, a death in the family or anything."

Jenny managed a giggle. "Goodness, no; nothing that serious. It's just that I lost my job and I'm pretty upset."

"That's good then. Not good that you lost your job, but good that no one died."

Jenny laughed in spite of herself. "You sound just like my Aunt Sue. When I told her, she shouted 'Congratulations!' at me."

"She seems to be a woman who knows what she's talking about. Why not congratulate yourself, by coming bowling with me and the kids? I've always found that one of the good things about losing something is that you either find it again, or replace it with something better. Someone as lovely and talented as you is bound to find a better job soon."

There was a pause. Jenny looked over at her aunt who was nodding violently with wide open eyes as if to say, "GO!"

"Seems like you need your mind made up for you," said Max. 'I'm going to pick you up in 30 minutes, then. See you soon!" With that, he hung up.

"Five, maybe six months, if I'm careful," Jenny said to Joy and her aunt as she hung up. "That's the answer to your earlier question about how long I could live relatively comfortably on my savings without a job."

"Wow, Jenny, that's quite a comfortable cushion. I had no idea you had saved so much," Joy patted her on the back, with obvious admiration.

"Actually, neither did I. I've never thought of my savings in terms of how long they could support me if I got laid off. I mean, how bad do you have to be to get laid off from higher education?" Jenny began to cry again. Joy handed her the glass of wine, but Jenny shook her head. "Dear old dad. He was the one who taught me early on that I should bank a quarter of my salary every paycheck. No exceptions. I guess it added up."

"So now that we've established that you're not going to starve or sleep in the park, at least for the short term - and with me and your aunt looking out for you, that would never happen anyway - the next step is to help you create a game plan," Joy said.

"Sure that's great. But can we do that tomorrow? I'm kind of talked out right now and besides, Max is on his way. We're going bowling." Jenny blew her nose and stood up, and headed toward her bedroom. "I'd better freshen up a bit." She looked directly at her aunt. "How bad do I look? Should I really be going on a date right now?"

"Best thing you could be doing. And you look fine," responded her aunt. "Splash some cold water on your face to counteract the puffiness. Use some of those eye drops I bought you for red eye, and come out of that room with a kick-ass attitude. Max will never know what hit him!"

"I agree," said Joy. "Best thing right now is to stop ruminating and do something fun and lighthearted." Joy squeezed Sue's arm affectionately. "And although I thought she had completely gone mad when she first said it, I agree with your aunt now that congratulations are in order! You've shifted so much recently that your current environment can no longer support you. It's time for a major life change. I'm excited for you."

Jenny retraced her steps and hugged her aunt and Joy. "Seriously, I don't know what I would do without the two of you. Thank you so much for being there for me. I love you both."

✳ ✳ ✳

"Glad to be going home?" Jenny asked her aunt as they stood in line at the airport, waiting to check in. "Say no and stay with me. You've become such an important fixture in my life … I don't think I can manage without you."

"That's exactly why this is the perfect time for me to leave," said Sue, pecking Jenny on the cheek. "That and the fact that I have two kitties who need rescuing from the boarders and friends who are asking where the heck I've disappeared to. I've got to get back to my normal life too, if you could ever call my life 'normal'."

"I'm scared," said Jenny, simply.

"Of your next adventure? I can't believe that! It's not change we fear, but the unknown that lies between what we're used to and what we really want. You'll be wandering around in 'no-person's land' for a little while, but you'll soon find your way. Just give yourself some space to decide what it is you want, then take some small incremental steps in any direction. Life will provide the signposts at the appropriate time," said Sue.

"And, remember we also have technology on our side. I'm just a phone call away. With Skype and Facetime, we can see each other as often as we'd like. Plus, you've promised to come visit me in a few weeks. I'm sending you the ticket. No arguments!"

"You know, you're right," said Jenny, feeling a sudden surge of confidence and excitement.

"Normally, right now, I'd be sitting at my desk doing work that didn't interest me, working for a man who is almost impossible to please, and going through the motions. It's great to wake up in the morning knowing that I have a whole day of discovery ahead of me!"

"That's my girl," said Sue, handing her flight itinerary to the airline staff. "And don't forget you've got Joy and Max supporting you every inch of the way. I'm so glad you met Max. He seems like a fun new friend. And that's the kind of person I think you need to be around right now, if you know what I mean."

Jenny gently punched her aunt's upper arm. "Now, auntie. I know you don't like Patty so much, but I've got that under control now. No more sitting around, moaning about the world, feeding our faces with fast food and pre-packaged junk. I have a pretty good picture of the life I intend to lead now. Patty is welcome to come along, but I'm not holding myself back to suit her."

Sue collected her boarding pass and heaved her luggage onto the conveyer belt.

"Fantastic! Sounds like you DO have everything under control! Okay, time for me to head for security. I'll call you when I get home. And I'll send you an email with all the details you need so you can meet with my friend who does the nutritional lab testing I was telling you about. Might as well do it while you're visiting me. She can help you identify the specific foods and nutrients that you need to pay attention to, so you can achieve your very best health and maximum energy levels. I found that to be a very important piece to my early journey. I still do follow-ups from time to time. There's no need to wait for my call if you and Max are planning anything. I'll just leave a voice message for you."

Sue hugged her niece affectionately. "Bye for now, my dear. Enjoy every step of your new life. I'm so proud of you!"

Jenny waved until her aunt disappeared from sight. She wiped a tear from the corner of her eye and turned to leave the airport. As she approached the exit doors, she caught sight of a slender silhouette in the glass.

Jenny stopped, and pulled out a compact mirror. While checking that her make-up wasn't smudged from crying, she held the mirror out, to look at her whole face.

"Well, there you are," she said to her reflection. "It's been a long time coming, but you've finally appeared. The woman I always knew I was meant to be. And, if I say so myself, you're looking pretty darn good."

And with that, Jenny strode confidently through the doors and into the warm morning air, smiling broadly.

CHAPTER 9

A New Beginning

"I can't believe how beautiful it is up here!" Jenny exclaimed, as she looked down over the valley from which they'd just climbed, and across the panorama that surrounded them. She dipped her celery stick into the pine nut garlic dip she'd made that morning, adding, "These kids are amazing. That was no easy climb! Had I not been training for the triathlon over the past few months, I'd never have made it myself."

Max laughed out loud. "There was never any doubt you'd get to the top Jenny, even if I had to throw you over my shoulder and carry you the rest of the way myself!" He poured smoothies for each of the kids while he finished making the sandwiches.

Jenny smiled as she realized how far she'd come in the past few months. A year ago, her Saturdays were spent on Patty's couch, stuffing her face with chips and dip, complaining about her life and yearning for something more. With a pang of sadness, she wondered how Patty was doing, and why her friend was so reluctant to change. Jenny had tried to include Patty in her new life, by inviting her to social events with Max and Joy, and the new friends she had made since leaving the university. Patty always found some excuse not to come. Then she stopped returning Jenny's calls, and they'd drifted apart. Jenny hadn't spoken to Patty in at least six months.

"I hope they like the drinks," Max called to Jenny, interrupting her thoughts. "Sadly, they're used to a lot of soda."

Jenny slowly stood up, rested and nourished, to help Max make lunch. She looked over at a group of young people were exchanging notes about their trip. Some were drawing, others were examining things they had collected along the hike, and a few were just sitting quietly, soaking in the beauty of nature. Each one of them looked so happy and connected. She smiled contentedly, beaming with pride at this group that she affectionately called "Max's Kids."

"Oh, they're going to love it!" said Jenny. "Aunt Sue taught me how to make them that specific way for kids and skittish adults. After I blended the frozen bananas and strawberries with fresh squeezed orange juice, I added a couple of small handfuls of spinach -- enough to boost the nutrition, but not so much to change the color to green. They won't even know there are greens in them!"

Max hugged Jenny and whispered in her ear, "Sneaky!" He turned his attention back to the task at hand. "What did you say was in the bread? It tastes an awful lot like rye."

"Mostly sprouted buckwheat, chia seed, and sunflower seeds, with a bit of onion and caraway seed. I added a couple of dates to keep it pliable, and then dehydrated it overnight. I learned how to do that in a class I took a couple of months ago, right before I got my food dehydrator ... which, I have to say, is my new best friend."

"I thought *I* was your new best friend," Max teased, squeezing Jenny's arm affectionately. "Don't tell me I got booted by a black box with a fan! And so soon into our relationship, too!"

Jenny kissed him on the cheek. "It's no ordinary black box, Max," she teased. "It's a magic black box that turns fresh vegetables and seeds into breads and crackers and pizza crusts!"

Max pulled one of his faces that Jenny found so adorable. "Hard to compete with magic," he said. "Especially when you can create such delicious bread without all that flour, sugar and oil. Tell me again why you think the kids shouldn't be eating gluten. I was trying to explain it to one of the volunteers the other day, and your eloquent explanation flew right out of my head."

After realizing that their shared passion was helping disabled kids discover education and career outcomes, Jenny developed a new program at the nonprofit where she now worked with Max. She'd had a feeling that there were some nutritional protocols they could apply, and had started researching which foods might enhance their physical and mental performance, rather than deplete their energy. Sure enough, she came across tons of information.

"Gluten has been associated with muscular dystrophy, balance problems, muscular degeneration and even paralysis. It messes up digestion, leaving sensitive people with poor nutrient absorption, which can lead to impaired growth and development."

Max laughed, gently punching Jenny's upper arm. "You sound like you swallowed a nutrition encyclopedia for breakfast," he joked.

Jenny looked around to be sure none of the kids were watching, and stuck out her tongue at him in mock annoyance. "Getting these kids away from bread and processed foods, and feeding them whole fresh fruits and veggies may not be the magic wand that makes all their challenges disappear, but it will improve the overall quality of their lives."

Max smiled at Jenny, beaming with pride at how seriously she was taking her commitment to his young charges. "Lunch is ready," he called to them, handing each of them a sandwich as they lined up before him.

Jenny sighed contentedly, as she helped Max pass out the food and drinks. She'd come to love these kids, and was enjoying her work with them more than she'd ever enjoyed anything she'd done before. What had really blown her away was how they were filled with optimism, joy and a determination to succeed, in spite of their physical and often mental challenges.

Shortly after she'd joined Max as a volunteer at New Start, helping to fill the time after being let go from her university job, a part-time position as the office manager had opened up. The timing was perfect. Jenny applied and was offered the job.

The small but steady income gave her plenty of free time to learn more about the value of good nutrition and, after sharing her knowledge with the nonprofit's executive director, they'd applied for - and received - a grant that they used to create a new position for her, so they could focus more on the overall health and well-being of the kids in their care.

A lot had happened since that day when Aunt Sue congratulated her for getting fired. Her aunt had been right after all about how, when you change from the inside, the external world changes too, to remain in alignment.

The sounds of nature were interrupted by the blare of Jenny's cell phone. "I can't believe there's a signal way out here in the middle of nowhere," said Jenny as she instinctively took the phone out of her pocket and glanced at the caller id. Jenny pressed the talk button. "Hi Joy."

"Jenny, I hate to bother you," said her friend on the other end of the line. "I know you're out on the big hike with Max's kids, but I'm so excited I can't contain myself! I was hoping you could pick up. Guess what?! I got it! That job I interviewed for. Remember? The one I really, really wanted? The one I thought was perfect for me? I got it!"

Jenny let out a scream of delight and gave a thumbs-up sign to Max, who was looking at her quizzically.

"I had my third interview yesterday, with the vice president!" Joy continued. "They'd narrowed it down to three candidates, and I was so nervous. They called me today to offer me the position. Can you believe that? On a weekend! But the HR woman said she didn't want to wait for the formal offer to make it through the process, in case I accepted another offer in the meantime. She was really impressed and wants me to start in two weeks, which is perfect for me. The bank requires two weeks' notice, so I won't have any downtime at all."

Joy paused to catch her breath and Jenny took the opportunity to congratulate her friend. "Joy, I'm so happy for you! What great news. I've been listening to you talk about this for weeks. It sounds like the perfect fit for your skills and your passion!"

Jenny smiled broadly, content at how everything was unfolding so beautifully. She wondered if Aunt Sue had any idea how many lives had been changed for the better, both directly and indirectly, by her influence. She'd probably shrug if Jenny brought it up to her. *Now, Jenny, you know it has very little to do with me. Everything you need is right here, inside you,* Jenny could almost hear her say. She felt as if her aunt's warm hand was placed over her heart even as she thought about her.

"Jenny, thanks so much for answering. I was about to burst with excitement, and I so wanted you to be the first to hear the news."

Jenny felt a rush of love and appreciation for her friend. Joy had been there for her through rough times as well as happy ones, and their increased closeness over the past ten months had been a constant source of comfort to her.

"Of course, Joy! I'm so thrilled for you! Gotta run now, sweetie," said Jenny. "We're just about to eat lunch, and I'm ravenous after our walk. Need to build up my energy for the long hike back down. Thanks so much for calling. I'll talk to you tomorrow."

Jenny smiled, and took a deep contented breath before joining the rest of the group for lunch.

The mock tuna sandwiches, brimming with sprouts and greens, were a big hit with the kids.

"This bread is different, but really awesome," one of them exclaimed. "The sandwiches my mom makes don't taste like much of anything at all, but I really like these."

Jenny beamed with pleasure. This was her first attempt at introducing healthier foods to the kids, and it seemed to be a big success so far.

Max reached out to Jenny, who was sitting on a rock at his side, and squeezed her shoulders. "Great job Jenny. And it sounds like Joy had some good news, too."

"Yes, she's been talking about wanting that job for weeks. She was so nervous before the last interview on Friday that she called me four times to rehearse!"

Max laughed. "I'm really happy for her. She's so gifted and passionate; I'm afraid she's been withering away at her current job."

Jenny reached up and squeezed Max's hand as it lay on her shoulder and thought how, not that long ago, she'd been in exactly the same position.

* * *

Jenny stood just outside the airport security gate, watching each face for the familiar sight of Aunt Sue. It had been nearly a year since she had stood in almost the same spot, scanning every frumpy gray haired woman who had walked past, in the hopes of recognizing her aunt. Now she knew differently.

Jenny was also very different from the overweight, unhappy and lonely figure who had awaited her aunt's arrival on that first occasion. Now she felt calm and confident, and she was proud of how polished she looked in her tight-fitting jeans and teal blue T-shirt Aunt Sue had sent her from one of her exotic trips. Jenny had noticed as she slipped into the shirt that morning how closely the color resembled Max's eyes.

"Max," she said under her breath. Just the mention of his name still made her tingly. She'd learned so much from him, not only about how work could be uplifting and purposeful, but about herself as well.

She and Aunt Sue would have about two weeks together before the big race. Jenny had been training for almost nine months and felt ready. "I doubt I'll be able to keep up with my aunt," she'd said to Max just the day before, "but at least I feel confident that I'll complete it, and maybe not come in dead last!"

Suddenly, Jenny spotted her aunt striding confidently toward the security gate, and her heart swelled with pride. *She's as beautiful as ever*, Jenny thought. This amazing woman was, to Jenny, a wizard, magician, loving mentor and friend. A catalyst for the change that had transformed her life!

The older woman raised a hand and waived at her niece. Jenny rushed through the crowd toward her. They fell into each other's arms and, ignoring everyone around them, stood for several minutes in a warm embrace.

"What's new?" asked her aunt when they had parted, and began walking together, arm-in-arm, toward the exit.

"How long do you have?" asked Jenny, beaming broadly.

YOUR Transformation Journey Toward Unstoppable Health

Throughout the book, we watched as Jenny went through the ups and downs - along with the joys and agonies - of incorporating a new and healthier diet and lifestyle. And maybe, just maybe, you can relate.

Jenny's story is not unique. It's similar to that of the many thousands of patients, clients and students I've counselled over the past 25 years. Did it sound familiar to you, as well?

How many times have you started a new diet or exercise program, only to "fall off the wagon" and have a hard time getting back on? Almost everyone I know, practitioners and clients alike, have had this experience.

Let's face it: We live in a world where healthy habits are the exception, not the norm, which can make the transition a challenge.

Knowing WHAT to do is an awesome start. Knowing HOW to create new habits that can be maintained - and that will become second nature - is where most people struggle. That's because it takes support, community, and accountability to really succeed.

I want you to know:

You Deserve Unstoppable Health

You were born to be healthy, and to have the energy, strength, and mental clarity to live a successful and joyful life.

Unfortunately, right from the start we are inundated with unhealthy habits and environments, from the bright lights and chemicals in the delivery room, to the formula, baby food, toxic baby care and cleaning products, and refined, sugar-laden foods we are fed as toddlers. We were, and mostly still are, surrounded by advertisements for foods devoid of nutrition, and drugs to get rid of the symptoms these foods create.

But right now, wherever you are in your life and whatever your state of health, you have the opportunity to turn it all around, and get yourself on the transformational journey toward Unstoppable Health.

As we learned through Jenny, food is just one of the factors crucial to stepping into a life of joy, vitality and fulfillment.

In fact, as part of my Nutritional Endocrinology™ approach, I teach the 7 Pillars of Unstoppable Health. When you master these 7 Breakthrough Habits, you *Feel Younger, Grow Stronger, and Enjoy More Energy* ... just as Jenny did.

Wondering what they are?

The 7 Breakthrough Habits:

1. Incorporate strategies to manage and transform stress.
2. Get in touch with what matters most, and keep it in your vision at all times.
3. Get deep and restful sleep.
4. Maintain nutritional balance by choosing whole, fresh foods.
5. Keep fit, by moving your body in ways you enjoy.

6. Clean up your environment, and get rid of toxic exposures.
7. Have fun – EVERY day!

Now, let's talk briefly about number 7, above.

Many people believe that having fun is mutually exclusive to eating a healthy diet and exercising regularly.

As Jenny discovered, making and eating nutritious foods can also be fun, pleasing to the palate *and* very rewarding, when it comes to both your physical appearance and your ability to do the things you like best.

Jenny also discovered that her new habits were much easier to continue with the support and guidance of Aunt Sue.

Perhaps right now you're thinking some (or all) of the following:

- "But I don't have an Aunt Sue."
- "This could never be me."
- "I'd love to experience this type of transformation, but I have no idea how or where to begin."
- "I already practice a lot of the habits Jenny adopts in the story, but I'm still not as energetic or healthy as I would like."

Wherever you are on your own health journey, if you're still not living with passion and purpose, awakening each day filled with energy and delicious anticipation about what the day holds in store for you, you could benefit from your own energy recharge!

When embarking on a health re-balancing journey like Jenny's, becoming a member of a community of likeminded people is essential, so you can get the support and encouragement you need when "the going gets tough."

It's also incredibly important to have an accountability system in place to keep you moving forward, which can also be provided by your fellow community members.

Finally, having a mentor you can trust (like Aunt Sue), who has your best interest at heart, and who is dedicated to keeping you pointed in the right direction is *invaluable*.

In fact, without a mentor or coach, it's like setting out on a journey with the destination in mind, but without a navigation system in place!

That's exactly why I'm giving you access to a wealth of FREE online support for your own Unstoppable Health Journey, so that you - like Jenny - can take powerful steps that lead you toward living your own passion and purpose.

That's right – I'm *giving* you the majority of the resources Aunt Sue mentions to Jenny, including a FREE copy of her "Healthy Eating-on-the-Run Survivors Guide," and all the yummy recipes she made!

And if you need an "Aunt Sue" to guide you, we can help with that too.

Go to http://www.UnstoppableHealthResources.com right now to download all our free resources, and to connect with a coach.

I hope you've enjoyed this book, and that you feel inspired to begin creating the lasting change that can – and will – transform your entire life!

All my best to you, on your journey toward Unstoppable Health.

Love, Unstoppable Health, and Joy,

Dr. Ritmarie Loscalzo

P.S. I'd LOVE for you to take a moment to share your thoughts about this book, and/or details about your own journey toward Unstoppable Health, with me on Facebook! Join us now, and connect with others who are on *their* own Unstoppable Health journeys, as well: http://www.drritamarie.com/go/UHRFacebook

P.P.S. If you are a health coach, nutritionist or other health practitioner, and you'd like to learn more about how you too can be at the forefront of Nutritional Endocrinology, visit http://www.nutritionalendocrinology.com

Summary of Key Takeaways

CHAPTER 3: A New Beginning

Wow – Aunt Sue taught Jenny so much in just a few hours together!

Here's a summary of what Jenny learned:

1. Water quality is important, and the kind of container you use matters! Always choose glass or metal.
2. Sea vegetables are loaded with minerals, and are especially important for your thyroid because of the iodine content, which is hard to find in other foods. Thyroid health is important for energy and metabolism, so you can more easily attain and maintain your ideal body weight.
3. A variety of greens is better than just using iceberg lettuce in salad, due to their high-nutrient density.
4. Eating late at night can contribute to feeling unrested in the morning, because your body is too busy digesting food to repair itself.
5. It's easy to make a quick, nutrient-dense meal that tastes great and satisfies.
6. You don't need to give up dessert to be healthy.

Action Steps:

Go back through the chapter to review the key take-aways listed above.

Visit www.UnstoppableHealthResources.com to download recipes, and get additional action steps and resources to motivate yourself to get into action.

Recipes in Chapter 3 include:

- Tropical Green Smoothie aka Quick Energy Drink
- Mock tuna
- Ginger Seaweed Salad
- Chocolate Mousse
- Nut Whipped Cream

CHAPTER 4: Change Is in the Air

Jenny is ready for change, and has learned so much already, in just one day with Aunt Sue.

Here's a summary of what Jenny learned:

1. The importance of emotional cleansing in regard to overall health and well-being – the necessity of getting out of emotionally draining and toxic situations and relationships in order to make positive, lasting change.
2. The importance of identifying what you most value and desire in your life, so you can live in alignment with those values and desires.
3. How to start slow with exercise, focusing on bursts of intensity, to build endurance.
4. How vitamin D deficiency can contribute to depression and loss of motivation, plus a host of other symptoms. Also, how to test for Vitamin D deficiencies, and the importance of spending time outdoors to replenish it.

Action Steps:

Go back through the chapter to review the key take-always listed above.

Visit www.UnstoppableHealthResources.com to download recipes, and get additional action steps and resources to motivate yourself to get into action.

Recipes in Chapter 4 include:

- Pina Colada Smoothie
- Apple Ginger Medley
- Nut Milk
- Tacos with romaine lettuce tortillas
- Guacamole
- Salsa
- Mock refried beans
- Apple pie

CHAPTER 5: The Slippery Slope

Yikes! Poor Jenny. After an amazing day complete with an accomplishment she could be proud of, Jenny rushes off to a party fraught with temptations. She does her best to control herself, and starts off with small bites of food and sips of wine. The addictiveness of her indulgences gets the better of her, and she finds herself sliding down a very slippery slope, feeling bloated, uncomfortable, and ultimately, like a hopeless failure.

Here's a summary of what Jenny learned:

1. Making healthy choices and eating before a party or event where enticing food abounds will help ward off temptation, so you can avoid sabotaging your best efforts.
2. It's virtually impossible to "eat just one." Comfort foods are addictive by nature, increasing your cravings.

Action Steps:

Visit www.UnstoppableHealthResources.com to download a special resource we've created to provide you with proven strategies for combatting emotional eating.

CHAPTER 6: Training Wheels

Jenny learned the importance of "training wheels" when it comes to adopting new habits and lifestyle changes. She discovers it's never a straight path. In the early stages especially, it's important to have a mentor or support system in place to guide you, and catch you when you fall. (And again, it's not "if" you fall, it's "when" - falling in the early stages is guaranteed to happen at least once!)

Action Steps:

Think about what matters most to you. What is the big WHY behind your desire to restore your energy, feel great and maintain your ideal weight? Write it down on an index card and carry it with you everywhere.

Then, visit www.UnstoppableHealthResources.com to download resources related to values and vision, as well as healthy travel and dining out tips.

CHAPTER 7: Race Day

Jenny is inspired and motivated by Aunt Sue's race, and by Max's dedication to a cause greater than himself. This motivates Jenny to get in touch with her own deepest desires, so she can work toward living a life of meaning and contribution.

Action Steps:

Consider your current job situation and ponder what you'd be doing instead, that would really fulfill you, if money was no object. Consider going through the same visualization process Jenny uses in this chapter, if you seek additional clarity.

Then, visit www.UnstoppableHealthResources.com to download recipes, and get additional action steps and resources to motivate yourself to get into action.

Recipes in Chapter 7 include:

- Superfood Energy Bars
- Race Day Green Juice
- Raspberry Orange Sorbet
- Low Glycemic No-Bake, Wheat Free Vanilla and Organic Chocolate "Cheese" Cake
- Chocolate Sauce

CHAPTER 8: A Blessing in Disguise

Jenny learns an important lesson when faced with what feels like a catastrophic event. She comes to realize that sometimes you need a bit of a push, when you're too scared to jump yourself ... and that what first appears as a crisis can actually be a gift in disguise.

Action Steps:

Think about a time in your life when an apparent catastrophe ended up becoming a turning point moment for you, instead.

Then, visit www.UnstoppableHealthResources.com to access additional resources and action steps.

CHAPTER 9: A New Beginning

YES!! Jenny has created lasting, positive change. She not only lands her dream job, but she has reached her goals of feeling confident, strong, and healthy

Action Steps:

Make a list of 5 steps you can begin taking right away – today - to move forward in the direction of your greatest dreams, goals, and visions.

Then, visit www.UnstoppableHealthResources.com to access additional recipes, resources, and action steps to help you put a plan in place.

Recipes in Chapter 9 include:

- Pine Nut Garlic Dip
- "Rye" Bread
- Onion Squash Bread
- Mock Tuna
- Mock Mayonnaise

About the Author

Dr. Ritamarie Loscalzo, MS, DC. CCN, DACBN

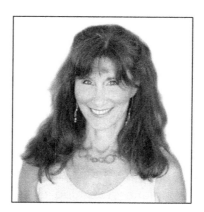

Dr. Ritamarie Loscalzo is passionately committed to transforming exhausted high-achievers all over the globe into high-energy people who love their lives and live to their full potential.

She founded the Institute of Nutritional Endocrinology so that she could be instrumental in transforming our current broken disease-management system into a true health care system, where each and every practitioner is skilled at finding the root cause of health challenges.

Dr. Ritamarie specializes in using the wisdom of nature married with modern scientific research to restore balance to hormones, with a special emphasis on thyroid, adrenal, and insulin imbalances. Her practitioner training programs empower health and nutrition experts - including coaches, physicians, nutritionists, nurses and others - to use functional assessments and natural therapeutics to unravel the mystery of their clients' complex health challenges, so they become known as go-to practitioners for true healing and lasting results.

Dr. Ritamarie is a licensed Doctor of Chiropractic with Certification in Acupuncture and is a Diplomat of the American Clinical Nutrition Board. She is a Certified Clinical Nutritionist with a Master of Science in Human Nutrition and Computer Science, and she has completed a 500-hour Herbal Medicine Certification Program.

Dr. Ritamarie is also certified as a living foods chef, instructor, and coach, and she has trained and certified hundreds of others in the art of using palate-pleasing, whole fresh food as medicine. As a certified HeartMath® provider, Dr. Ritamarie is passionate about using HeartMath® stress transformation techniques to guide clients to reduce the negative impact of stress on their health.

Her passion for health and healing began as a result of her own bout with illness. After recovering her health by changing how and what she ate, along with how she actually lived her life, Dr. Ritamarie began her formal training in nutrition and natural medicine in 1985.

When she's not writing, speaking, or coaching around health and nutrition topics, Dr. Ritamarie loves to run, hike, swim, paint, make pottery and travel with her husband and two vibrant and active sons.

Dr. Ritamarie can be reached at www.DrRitamarie.com.

To find out more about her programs for health and wellness professionals, visit www.NutritionalEndocrinology.com.

Other Books by Dr. Ritamarie Loscalzo

Trendsetters Trend Setters - Chapter 39, Adrenal Recharge
Strategies for High Achievers

One Crazy Broccoli Chapter 26: Unlocking My Inner
Healer
and My Journey to Health and Joy

Assess Your Own Body Chemistry

Blended Greens for Health and Longevity

Blitz That Belly

Creating a Healing Kitchen

Deliciously Quick Lunch and Dinner

Desserts: Making It Rich Without Oil (co-author)

Dried and Gone to Heaven (co-author)

Eliminate the Gluten and Accelerate Your Health

Made in the USA
Coppell, TX
22 April 2021